D0938240

Epidemic of Care

George C. Halvorson
George J. Isham

· ·

Foreword by
Alain Enthoven

Epidemic of Care

- -

A Call for Safer, Better, and More Accountable Health Care

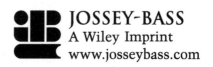
JOSSEY-BASS
A Wiley Imprint
www.josseybass.com

Published by Jossey-Bass
A Wiley Imprint
989 Market Street, San Francisco, CA 94103-1741   www.josseybass.com

Jossey-Bass books and products are available through most bookstores. To contact
Jossey-Bass directly call our Customer Care Department within the U.S. at 800-956-7739,
outside the U.S. at 317-572-3986, or fax 317-572-4002.

Jossey-Bass also publishes its books in a variety of electronic formats. Some content that
appears in print may not be available in electronic books.

Library of Congress Cataloging-in-Publication Data

Halvorson, George C.
Epidemic of care : a call for safer, better, and more accountable health care / George C.
Halvorson and George J. Isham.
p. cm. —
Includes bibliographical references and index.
ISBN 0-7879-6888-9 (alk. paper)
1. Health care reform—United States. 2. Health Care Costs—United States.
3. Health Services Accessibility—United States. 4. Insurance, Health—economics—
United States. 5. Medically Uninsured—United States.
I. Isham, George J. II. Title.
RA395.A3 H3448 2003
WA 540 AA1 H118e 2003
362.1/0425 21
                                    2003002583

Printed in the United States of America
FIRST EDITION
HB Printing   10 9 8 7 6 5 4 3 2

Contents

. . . .

Preface and Acknowledgments

. . . .

For nearly a decade, we worked as a team at HealthPartners to improve the quality and affordability of health care in Minnesota. We were partners in dozens of efforts aimed at making health care more accountable and accessible. This book represents what we believe to be true about reforming and improving both the financing and delivery of care.

It describes why health care costs are going up, who is accountable for those cost increases, and what can be done to make care significantly better.

We now work for separate organizations, but we continue to share a commitment to care improvement and widespread understanding of the key issues. This book is an extension of that old partnership to a new set of efforts—and to create a more informed national dialogue on these key issues.

We would like to acknowledge the leadership of the Health-Partners board of directors and the thinking of Don Berwick, John Wennberg, Peggy O'Kane, Alain Enthoven, Uwe Reinhard, Paul Ellwood, Mary Brainerd, and the new leadership colleagues at Kaiser Permanente in helping develop the perspectives outlined in this book.

We are grateful to Maureen Peterson, who has helped us organize this effort and keep track of a tremendous amount of information.

We are also grateful to Nancy Langer who has typed many drafts of this book, often from very nearly illegible handwritten notes.

February 2003   GEORGE C. HALVORSON
                                             Oakland, California

                                             GEORGE J. ISHAM
                                             Minneapolis, Minnesota

Foreword

Health insurance premiums, currently increasing about 15 percent per year, are on a track to double in five years. If this goes on much longer, the result will be a financial catastrophe for patients, doctors, nurses, administrators, pharmaceuticals, medical device manufacturers, insurers, employers, and everyone else touched by our health care system.

Perhaps you're thinking, "This isn't news." After all, our country has been through this before; we'll get through it again. But there is indeed something quite new and different about today's health cost crisis, as George Halvorson and Dr. George Isham point out in this exceptionally clear and readable book.

In the past, these percentage increases took place on top of a much lower base. When the average family premium was $2,000 a year, a 15 percent increase meant an additional $300 per year. That wasn't a great deal as a percentage of total compensation. But now, as family premiums approach $10,000 a year and more, a 15 percent increase is an additional $1,500 per year, an amount likely to consume all, most of, or more than the increase in total compensation that employers can afford for many employees. Even on top of an *average* employee health benefit cost of about $6,500 in 2003, a 15 percent increase means an additional $975 per year.

Consider this example. An employee's total compensation is $40,000 in pay and $10,000 in employer-paid health insurance. An employer can afford to pay, in total compensation, no more than the value of the employee's contribution to the output of the firm. A policy of paying more than the value of employees' contributions means reduced profits, angry shareholders (including retirees' pension funds), and a call for new management.

Like many other employers, this company can afford raises in total compensation of no more than 3 percent for inflation and productivity. That's $1,500. Meanwhile, health insurance premiums rise by 15 percent. The premium increase consumes the raise. If this process continues, something will have to give. The employer will have to require the employee to contribute to the premium, or cut back on coverage, or cut pay, or lay off employees, or close the plant and move to a less costly area and possibly quit providing health insurance altogether. Meanwhile, employees who recently demanded an end to the restrictions of managed care now want to know the reason that their premium costs are up and their pay is down. As I write, General Electric employees are striking over this issue. As you read this, more workers will be threatening strikes.

The government's story is similar. About 60 percent of the health care bill in the United States is a cost to government budgets, including Medicare, Medicaid, the Veterans Administration, county hospitals, public employees' health care, and large tax breaks for employer-paid health insurance. Rising health costs are hitting government hard at a time of low revenue growth, forcing consideration of drastic cuts in education, criminal justice, public safety, and other programs. Higher taxes are no solution. Americans have a limited tolerance for taxes. In 2000, both presidential candidates found it in their electoral interest to propose tax cuts. So as a nation, rising health care expenditures are driving us to some painful choices: cut vital programs, raise taxes, or get serious about understanding and correcting the major flaws in our costly, unsafe, and inconsistent health care nonsystem.

It is easier to look for villains than for solutions. Pick your villain: greedy pharmaceutical companies, insurance companies, hos-

pital monopolies, overpaid doctors, unions or trial lawyers, or bureaucracy. It couldn't possibly be our unreasonable demands and expectations of our health care system.

Meanwhile, politicians circle the scene and look for partisan advantage by offering simplistic solutions: price controls, or a single
payer as in Canada or the United Kingdom, where everybody is
covered and health spending is low. Then some go to those countries. They see long waiting times, crumbling nineteenth-century
buildings, and deprivation of the technologies we take for granted,
and they lose enthusiasm. Others engage in magical thinking.

There is no single villain responsible for our troubles and no silver bullet to cure them. The sad thing is that very few people have
thought carefully and deeply about the problem, or understand what
is going on and where constructive solutions can be found.

To this scene, Halvorson and Isham bring to bear unusually
powerful and well-informed insight into the causes of these problems, combined with great clarity of exposition. The causes they
describe are many and complex. Their list includes many costly
medical miracles, free access to which everyone feels entitled; an
unsafe, error-prone system that, as often as not, fails to deliver effective and appropriate care; a widespread belief in entitlement to
unproven experimental care and care of very low marginal value
compared to its extra cost; a failure to do proper evaluations of new
technologies before general use; irresponsible politicians who pass
laws mandating the coverage of extremely costly but unevaluated
treatments (some of which turn out to be worthless or harmful);
local care monopolies created by mergers of most of the hospitals
or most of the doctors in town in a single specialty; a system that
creates cost-unconscious demand for new drugs, permitting drug
companies to charge ten times the price for the new drug that is
only marginally better than the old one; high, rising, and unreal-
istic patient expectations; serious shortages of nurses and other
technically trained personnel, the solution to which will have to
include large pay increases; and the relaxation of managed care cost

controls forced by the anti–managed care backlash and its accompanying lawsuits.

There is no doubt that American medical care today can confer many large benefits that were not available ten or twenty years ago. This is wonderful, and we should all be grateful for it. But there can also be no doubt that our lack of organized delivery systems working systematically to improve quality and value, our lack of incentives for economical choices all around, and our lack of a national health policy to guide the system cause our health care to cost much more than it needs to.

The authors recommend seven fundamental, practical strategies based on their and others' successful innovations. Halvorson and Isham have personally led many of the innovations they describe, and their recommendations are well grounded in experience. They know what they're talking about.

This book is comprehensive, thorough, practical, and very readable. As an economist, I particularly appreciated the authors' ability to grasp and explain the economic issues. Everyone with a serious interest in American health care must read this book. As we seek to move the national dialogue to a higher level, this book will be an invaluable guide.

Stanford, California   ALAIN ENTHOVEN
February 2003   Marriner S. Eccles Professor of Public
                                              and Private Management (Emeritus)
                                                     Graduate School of Business,
                                                              Stanford University

Introduction

. . . .

What Happened to My Paycheck?

Health care costs are exploding in America. Right now, health care consumes 14 percent of the gross national product (GNP).[1] If the current rate of cost increase continues and the economy continues to falter, health care could actually consume 20 percent of the GNP within five years.[2] That will be triple the projected average level of health care expenditures in other industrialized countries. Health care premiums in the United States are now going up from 12 to 20 percent a year (depending on the market), and with no break in sight. Premium increases of 30 to 40 percent are not unheard of for some insurers and some customers.

The impact of those cost increases on both employers and employees will be huge. American workers will see a direct cut in their take-home pay over the next two years. Additional millions will lose health insurance coverage altogether. Many senior citizens, living on what they had hoped would be fixed incomes, are going to be particularly hard hit, with premiums for their Medicare supplement plans (and prescription drug costs) skyrocketing as their monthly income deteriorates due to stock market downturns that have seriously damaged retirement nest eggs.

Upset and angry voters of all ages will demand solutions from our politicians, and our politicians will find themselves trapped in a political nightmare.

Those policymakers who have spent the past five years cele-
brating the passage of laws whose direct and immediate impact has
been to expand health care spending will very soon be forced to rethink their positions. However, their initial solutions may well leave
quite a bit to be desired. The first round of political response will
probably be aimed at finding villains, punishing wrongdoers, and
simplistically assigning blame. As you will read in this book, that
approach will not solve the problems. The real issues are not hard
to understand, but they are going to take a much higher level of
strategic thinking to resolve.

At this stage of the health care economy, we need better leadership than we've had on these issues. Rhetoric will not rebuild paychecks. The politically expedient health care speeches of the last
decade won't be relevant for the problems of this decade. What will
be relevant will be shrinking paychecks and angry voters looking
for someone to blame.

Why will Americans' take-home pay go down?

Because employers will stop absorbing the full cost increases in
health care premiums.

Today's huge health care cost increases are already causing significant expense problems for many American companies. Employers provide most health care coverage in this country. They are now
facing some tough choices. Employers that decide simply to absorb
the exploding costs and pay the full health care premium increases
for their employees will either be forced to increase the price of
their own products (making them potentially less competitive), or
they will see a direct decrease in their corporate profits. A significant profit drop could have a negative impact on stock prices, an
unacceptable option for quite a few companies. The economy has
already taken a number of blows. Cutting profits significantly to buy
health insurance for employees will not seem like the best strategy
for either stockholders or senior management for many companies.
So to protect both profits and stock prices, most employers will figure out some way to shift or eliminate those additional costs.

While the U.S. economy was strong and we were in a very tight employment market, most employers did bite the bullet and simply picked up the increased health care expense for their employees.

Those days are rapidly ending. Employers in all areas of the economy, including the government, are now looking for expense cuts, not major expense increases.

How will employers cut their health care costs? Some employers, primarily smaller companies, will drop coverage altogether. Most employers, however, will shift costs of health coverage directly to their employees—by reducing the level of insurance benefits or forcing individual employees to pay a larger part of the premium.

Each of these inevitable cost-shifting decisions will make people unhappy. In combination, they have the potential to create a major political backlash. People who would not have considered the possibility of supporting a single-payer government-run system will now begin to wonder whether the private sector has failed entirely and a government-run solution is needed. Employers will also increasingly wonder whether a government-run system might have a lesser negative impact on the corporate expense budgets. Even state governments, faced with huge spending deficits for both Medicaid and employee health care, will consider whether it might just be easier to transfer the entire burden back to the federal government through some kind of single-payer system. In the short term, many states are simply cutting back on their Medicaid programs. California alone will cut nearly 500,000 people from that program in the next year.

The Upcoming Political Backlash Will Be Huge

But before employers turn to the government for a long-term answer, they will take the initial step of shifting costs to deal with today's problem.

It's hard to blame them for that decision. Health care premiums used to be a small portion of an employer's expense burden. Not any more. For a great many employers, the cost of a family premium for relatively full coverage is now running roughly $800 a month per employee, not a lot less than the minimum wage for a full-time worker. (The minimum wage now is $893 a month. Health care costs will exceed that in about two years at the current rate of increase.)

A 20 percent increase in premium costs moves that $800 per month family premium up to $960 per month. If current trends continue, then in year two, a second 20 percent increase will push up the premium to over $1,150 per month. That's a huge additional per employee expense for employers to absorb.

Most employers that face cost increases of that magnitude won't simply absorb those new costs. They will shift them to employees. That direct cost shift will have a shocking impact on the take-home pay of American workers.

A 12 Percent Premium Increase Wipes Out a 4 Percent Salary Increase

Consider the company with the $800 family premium. If that employer decides to freeze corporate contributions at current levels for two years, then the full $350 a month in higher premiums would have to come directly out of each worker's paycheck. Think about the impact of a $350 cut in monthly take-home pay for the average American. That's a $4,200 reduction in annual take-home pay for the average worker.

That cut in pay will cause a level of economic unhappiness for working Americans unrivaled by any other single issue in the past two decades. The $350 per month cut in individual take-home pay far eclipses the relatively tiny $350 a year tax rebates promoted so enthusiastically by our politicians just a couple of years ago.

If you optimistically assume that health care premium increases for the next couple of years can be held to a relatively low level, say 12 percent, the impact is still painful. Even a 12 percent increase in health care premium makes a 4 percent salary raise completely disappear for the average nonmanagement worker. No one is predicting premium increases of less than 12 percent for the next several years. Take-home pay will shrink for millions of Americans.

Politicians won't be alone in having to deal with the backlash from that explosion in costs. Labor leaders will be forced into some very difficult positions. They are already being faced with immense pressure from their members relative to health care costs.

Insurance cost subsidies could very quickly rise to the top of organized labor's priority list for negotiations and will probably become a strike issue in many settings. We've seen that happen already in local negotiations in a number of markets.

Workers in the 1990s Got to Keep Their Raises

Over the past decade, a number of factors outlined in some detail later in this book held health care costs relatively flat, a blessing for American workers. Because costs were flat, workers in the 1990s got to keep their raises. That issue isn't often discussed in the great debate about managed care in America, but the mathematics that prove that case are pretty easy to do. Private sector health care cost controls and various managed care approaches let real income and actual take-home pay grow for most American consumers.

No more.

Many of the controls that worked in the 1990s are no longer able to hold care costs in check. New laws and regulations compiled with new negotiating power gained by America's caregivers have undermined the leverage of health plans and insurers to the point where many of the same pressures that created double-digit health care inflation in the 1980s are now raising their expensive heads again.

The New Uninsured Will Also Be Voters— and Much Harder to Ignore

If the economy weakens even more than it has, the problem could get a lot worse. Senior citizens with diminished investment incomes will find Medicare supplemental coverage unaffordable and stand-alone

Medicare benefits to be inadequate and unacceptable. Millions of additional Americans will lose their coverage altogether. If current surveys are accurate about the likelihood of small employers dropping health insurance completely (if they face consecutive 15 to 20 percent annual premium increases), then 10 to 20 million additional working Americans could suddenly find themselves with no coverage at all over the next two to three years.[3]

The anger of the people who end up with smaller paychecks will be compounded by the outrage of the newly uninsured. The size of our uninsured population will, for the first time in recent memory, become a real political issue in America.

Up to now, the high number of uninsured Americans has not truly been a hot political pressure point. It has often been the subject of energetic rhetoric, but actually fixing the problem has never been the object of sufficient political consensus or energy to result in a legislative solution.

Except for the attempts at health care reform by President Bill Clinton and Hillary Clinton in 1992 and 1993, it has been far too easy for politicians to ignore the 42.1 million Americans who are uninsured because most of the permanently uninsured have not been voters. Therefore, politicians could all safely pretend they didn't exist. The small subset of the uninsured population who usually votes are mostly people who are only temporarily uninsured, that is, individuals in transition between jobs or between education and employment. They tend to be uninsured for a very short time, so they typically aren't particularly upset about being uninsured. Most expect to have coverage soon. Many still have COBRA (Consolidated Omnibus Budget Reconciliation Act of 1985) coverage, federal legislation that temporarily extends eligibility for group coverage as a transition safety net. Politicians therefore don't hear from the current permanent or temporarily uninsured population in any persuasive way. It hasn't been a voter issue.

That will now change.

In stark contrast, we believe the next large wave of uninsured people will be politically active. If, in fact, another 10 million or so working Americans find themselves uninsured over the next couple of years, their voices will be heard. These newly uninsured Americans will be a different category of citizenry: solidly and continuously employed people who suddenly find themselves totally without a health care safety net because of soaring health care premium costs. These people will be voters, and they will not be happy. Politicians will hear from the new uninsured. They will want answers and solutions.

In other words, we are on the verge of a whole new era of health care politics. It's time to face reality and recognize that we are moving into a major health care crisis in this country, driven by the way we deliver, receive, and pay for care.

Interestingly, there is both good news and bad news in the total health care picture.

The Health Care Tool Kit Gets Better Every Day

The good news in health care is how much it has improved. New drugs ease pain, reduce depression, control cholesterol, manage hypertension, improve sexual function, and generally make life more livable for millions of Americans. New technologies quiet tremors, replace failed joints, keep diseased hearts beating, and hunt down errant cancer cells. New scanning procedures allow physicians to view the body through incredible imaging technology that feels as much like magic as science.

Every single one of those new and wonderful care improvements costs money, and most cost a lot of money. The public appetite for better technology, better drugs, and better care is almost insatiable. The new approaches get purchased and used, so our engineers, inventors, and manufacturers are lined up to develop more devices, techniques, and drugs as quickly as possible. The two most profitable aspects of health care in this country today are prescription drugs and medical technology.

As new procedures and technologies become available, there is great pressure on insurers to pay for them all, often before the testing is complete to see if the new techniques or processes even work. There are no significant economic brakes, public or private, applied at any point to the introduction of new treatments, new drugs, new technology, or new procedures into American health care.

In stark contrast to the rest of the industrialized world, where government forces consistently work strategically to keep health care costs down, the actions of our lawmakers have strongly encouraged the current American cost trend. Instead of trying to slow health care cost increases, our legislators regularly pass laws and our regulators routinely enact edicts to mandate expanding the scope of both insurance benefits and health care services available to insured citizens. Literally thousands of those laws have been passed across the country. The trend of those particular laws is pretty clear. Less than one-tenth of 1 percent of the health care laws in the country in the past decade were written to limit any benefit or to require that real value, efficacy, or usefulness standards be applied to any type of new care.

Why? Because the public wants unlimited care. Voters want unlimited care. Patients definitely want unlimited care. So the constant, unspoken, but consistently followed public policy of this country has been to encourage insurance benefits that pay for unlimited health care for all American citizens who are fortunate enough to have private health coverage.

In the 1990s, when a number of factors described later in this book worked to keep overall health care cost trends down, that public policy agenda made sense. When costs are flat, expanding coverage seemed like a very reasonable political agenda. Everyone in politics got on that bandwagon.

What's a Better Use of Our Money Than Health?

Our clear expectation as a society and as a country now is that everyone who has insurance should get all of the care that he or she wants or could possibly use. That's not necessarily a bad standard to follow. Health is valuable. Being healthy is a good thing to be.

What's a better use of any nation's economic strength than providing care and improved health to its citizens? If we're going to spend the GNP on something, why not spend it on curing cancer and replacing hips rather than purchasing faster modems or upgrading computer chips? If forced into a real choice, why not spend our money on restoring hearing, repairing vision, or improving mobility rather than driving bigger cars, paving farmland to build wider highways, or developing ever more deadly laser-targeted missiles or undetectable plastic landmines? We will spend the GNP on one thing or another. Why not choose health?

Health is, beyond any doubt, an invaluable asset for both individuals and society at large, so why not make complete and comprehensive care available to all citizens? Who can argue against that goal?

Inconsistent, Wasteful, and Unaccountable Care

Unfortunately, the somewhat hypocritical, perversely incented, and frequently dysfunctional ways we've chosen to accomplish that goal as a country has left us with over 40 million uninsured citizens, amazingly inconsistent and unaccountable care, and the fastest-growing and most wasteful health care delivery economy in the world.[4] We are already paying for a lot more care than we are getting because large segments of our care system are stunningly inefficient and rigidly unfocused. Major portions of our health care delivery system are also unsafe.

Our health care delivery system in the United States is really a nonsystem with millions of independent, uncoordinated, separately motivated moving parts, each with its own economic priorities and self-focused financial goals. To quote Margaret O'Kane, president of the National Committee for Quality Assurance, "American health care has no central nervous system." No one in the overall system coordinates the overall patterns of care. No one develops and implements overall strategies for improving population health. No one measures, records, and reports comparative quality levels or care outcomes at the caregiver level. In almost all settings, each individual health care business entity—each doctor, hospital, pharmacy, surgery center, and so on—focuses on its own individual billable units of care and develops its own individual strategies. Too often, those strategies are aimed at maximizing each provider's market share, cash flow, and profitability rather than on improving service and creating more effective patient-centered approaches to care.

Our current incident-based, fee-paid, uncoordinated approach to care creates constantly expanding costs, an outcome that should surprise no one who understands economics, financial incentives, or production processes at any level.

We get what we pay for. There are over eight thousand separate billing codes set up for various units of care.[5] There isn't one single billing code set up for a cure. There is no fee for preventing a disease. The system does what it is paid to do. That really shouldn't surprise anyone.

Now we are finding ourselves as a nation in a truly difficult position. The massive and unrelenting increases in health care costs are going to make a great many people very angry in the very near future. No one in a position of policy leadership or authority currently has the power, leverage, legal status, skills, perspective, or database needed to make the current nonsystem produce more care for less money.

Few policymakers and even fewer citizens understand how badly the overall health care delivery system functions when it comes to incenting or encouraging efficiency and improving resource utilization. As a consequence, only a very tiny percentage of the population has any sense at all of why health care costs are going up.

Massive Finger Pointing Is the Logical Next Step

Although the public has little sense of the underlying reasons for the cost increases and no sense of what range or set of solutions is possible, anyone who knows basic human nature can predict that when personal paychecks get cut for millions of Americans and insurance disappears entirely for millions more, the public will very soon want someone or something to blame.

That's just a natural and normal human reaction. When things go wrong, there's a natural tendency to identify villains—to ferret out and punish wrongdoers. There's an equally powerful natural tendency when times are tough to initially seek out simplistic solutions—silver bullets—that can offer the illusion of solving a problem without anyone having to diagnose or manage the real factors that are causing that problem. Public thinking about health care seems to be particularly susceptible to that kind of response.

So what's next? Count us as cynics—and optimists.

As the current crisis unfolds, we expect massive finger pointing. We can count on punitive but misguided legislation. We can count on almost frenzied levels of political gamesmanship by far too many parties.

We can also count on a groundswell of enthusiasm for a government-run care system—that is, until journalists, consumer activists, and policymakers visit a few of those systems and get a close look at how those government-run systems actually operate. Before that happens, we can count on "single payer" becoming a war cry for a wide array of interests and groups.

What we hope for, but cannot count on, is an informed debate about the entire topic of our nation's health care system with all the facts and all of the relevant information out on the table for all to see.

That's too bad, because we are rapidly nearing a point where real choices need to be made. The actual care trends need to be understood. We need to know where solutions are desirable and, more important, where they are possible. We also need to face facts. Drug costs will continue to rise. So will technology costs. So will physician fees and hospital bills. Our population will continue to age. We need to recognize that our citizenry is increasingly both obese and inert. We need to understand the importance of the amazing fact that the number of diabetics in this country has gone up by over 33 percent since 1990 alone, a fact that shouldn't surprise anyone since the number of middle-aged Americans who are definably obese increased from 14.4 percent in 1982 to 26.7 percent in 1999.[6]

Diabetes is a disease that can be prevented in most people by physical activity and a healthy diet. Instead, our population has chosen dangerous eating patterns and behaviors that now have diabetics using nearly 25 percent of all dollars spent by Medicare.[7] The long-term consequences of just that one disease are devastatingly expensive. Other diseases are following similar patterns. Amazingly, almost no one is looking at those patterns. No one is discussing them in public forums. The public doesn't even know these extremely expensive and damaging problems of public health exist.

As a result of all those factors hitting us at the same time, health care costs are skyrocketing. Unless the actual cost drivers are clearly understood, there's little likelihood of avoiding intensive public anger and no likelihood of avoiding additional cost increases for our citizens and both our private and governmental payers.

Unless the health care delivery system goes through an extensive reengineering to take full and consistent advantage of science-based, outcomes-focused, computer-supported medical best practices, we will continue to see an epidemic of dysfunctional care and care outcomes that fall far below what we deserve and what we are paying for.

There are answers, but they aren't easy ones. The answers will take very bright people working hard to reengineer major aspects of health care to make it more patient centered and science based. We also need to follow the lead of every other profession and use the computer to augment the professional skills, memory, and performance of our caregivers. Those sound like the logical things to do, but those key steps are an extremely large challenge and will require enlightened buyers, care providers, policymakers, and patients. For starters, we need to understand the issues.

That's why we wrote this book. This book is intended to offer an overview of the major problems in health care today. It's a primer on health care cost drivers. It's written for the American worker whose salary increase for 2002 was just wiped out entirely by an increase in health care premium costs. It's also written for the legislator or policymaker whose job will be to deal with that angry worker.

This book was written to help create an informed debate. Unless we understand the entire system, we have no hope of fixing it. We offer some practical, field-tested, possibly controversial suggestions about how to make health care in the United States more accountable, more efficient, more valuable, and more affordable. If nothing else, we hope *Epidemic of Care* will start some interesting conversations.

This book is dedicated to
George Isham's father, Dr. William H. Isham
and
George Halvorson's four sons: Jonathan, Seth,
Charles, and Michael

The Authors

. . . .

George C. Halvorson is the chairman and chief executive officer for Kaiser Permanente, the nation's largest nonprofit health care delivery system. This multispecialty, group practice, prepayment program provides or arranges for members' care, including preventive services, routine and specialty care, hospital services, and pharmacy services. It serves more than 8 million members in nine states and the District of Columbia.

Before joining Kaiser Permanente, Halvorson served as the chief executive officer of several health plans, with his longest tenure as president and chief executive officer of HealthPartners in Minnesota.

Halvorson has been involved in health plan senior leadership in the United States since the mid-1970s and has also helped start health maintenance organizations in Uganda, Jamaica, and Spain. He has been the chair of the American Association of Health Plans, the Group Health Association of America, the Healthcare Education and Research Foundation, the American Diabetes Association's Managed Care Committee, and the hospital safety coalition Safest in America. He is currently vice chair for both the International Federation of Health Plans and the Alliance of Community Health Plans.

Among his books on health care–related topics, *Strong Medicine* is his most recent. He currently serves on the Commonwealth Fund

Task Force on the Future of Health Insurance and is a member of the Harvard/Kennedy School Healthcare Delivery Policy Program.

George J. Isham is medical director and chief health officer for HealthPartners, a nonprofit family of Minnesota health care organizations focused on improving the health of its members, its patients, and the community. It provides health care services, insurance, and health coverage to nearly 670,000 members. HealthPartners includes Group Health, founded in 1957, and Regions Hospital, an affiliate since 1993.

Isham is active in strategic planning and policy issues as well as quality and medical management. He is responsible for health promotion and disease prevention, research, and health professionals' education at HealthPartners.

Isham is a founding board member of the Institute for Clinical Systems Improvement, a collaborative of Twin Cities medical groups and health plans that is implementing clinical practice guidelines in Minnesota. He serves as cochair of the National Committee for Quality Assurance's committee on performance measurement, which oversees the national quality measurement standard for health plans (HEDIS). He is a founding member of the advisory board for the National Guideline Clearinghouse and a member of the Centers for Disease Control and Prevention's Task Force on Community Preventive Services. He has served on the Institute of Medicine's Board on Health Promotion and Disease Prevention and has served on a number of IOM committees.

He received his master of science in preventive medicine/administrative medicine from the University of Wisconsin-Madison and his doctor of medicine from the University of Illinois-Chicago.

Epidemic of Care

. . . .

Miracles Cost Money

Modern medical technology can keep tiny, fragile, extremely premature babies weighing only a pound alive. Modern medical technology can then provide lifetime services to even the smallest of these premature infants, many of whom have permanently underdeveloped lungs, inadequate kidneys, and, in some cases, lifelong brain function difficulties. A decade ago, these tiniest children would have died. Today, we can perform miracles.

Those miracles cost money. And sometimes those miracles can cost money for a very long time. The cost of prolonging many lives for long periods of time is a relatively new factor in health care expenses. Very sick people used to die. Now, many partially recover— and become permanent patients of one kind or another.

Being a permanent patient used to be a rare event. When kidney dialysis was invented to keep people with failed kidneys from dying, the actuaries who predicted future insurance costs were completely off the mark on their expense projections for kidney patients. They very accurately predicted the cost differences for the first year by adding up the new treatment costs for all of the kidney dialysis patients who would otherwise have died that year. What the actuaries forgot to take into account, however, was that most of the dialysis patients were now going to live for many additional years. The actuaries were accustomed to a world in which all kidney failure patients died relatively quickly. So the actuaries simply did one-year noncumulative expense projections. The total annual costs of treating all patients with failed kidneys turned out to be, in just a few years, four to five times higher than the actuaries had initially projected.

Saving those lives is a great accomplishment. It is truly miraculous, in fact, that dialysis could so successfully prolong lives. That is particularly wonderful news for the dialysis patients. The long-term costs, however, were a real shock to the people pricing health insurance. A powerful lesson was revealed about projecting the full long-term cost impact of specific new technologies. Only a few health insurance actuaries, however, learned that lesson. It was invisible to the public.

New technologies can improve health, improve functioning, and make life a lot better for patients in many areas. And the cumulative impact of all of those technologies puts a huge relatively new cost burden on the overall system.

The public at large remains ignorant of that cost impact. We see the impact of that miraculous care on individual patients' lives, but no one talks in any useful way about the impact of that miraculous care on cumulative community health care costs. Because no one ever presents the cost data to the public, the American people believe that today's medical miracles are free. They're not.

We are fortunate to live in a world where care is improving every day. Almost without exception, each improvement is more expensive than the care it replaces. In many instances, better care keeps people alive longer and, as a result, prolongs the time in which those people will receive care and incur expenses.

It can easily cost a million dollars to save a one-pound premature baby from death. If that child turns out to be permanently physically impaired, it can then cost anywhere from $50,000 to $200,000 annually to keep that child alive.[1] It will often take lifelong medical support services to provide each impaired child with acceptable levels of function and interaction. Each life saved is a miracle. The cost impact of those miracles is cumulative. One such child might cost $200,000 a year. Five similar cases then might cost a given community, in total, a million dollars a year for maybe fifty years. Let's say that we add ten such children every year to a local health care expense pool. Do the math. It's fascinating.

What's even more fascinating is that no one actually does the math. These cost issues are invisible.

When the famous McCaughey septuplets were born in 1997, one part of the story that was almost totally ignored or overlooked by the news media was the cost of the care needed to keep those babies alive. Conservatively, total expenses incurred in helping those seven tiny babies survive to their first birthday exceeded $2 million.

That was money well spent. All seven of those babies seem to have benefited immensely from the wonderful care they received. Miracles were accomplished. We Americans are very good at those miracles.

Nowhere else in the world would the odds have been in favor of all seven of those babies living to see their first birthday—or even in favor of all seven babies living for a full week after their birth. We truly do miracles here. Those miracles cost money. None of the news stories about those babies bothered to total up the costs. To the public, the McCaughey miracle seemed to be free, a gift, maybe, from the care system. Not true. Bills were incurred. An insurer paid those bills. Millions of dollars changed hands: $2 million just for starters.

Premature infants tend to be some of the more extreme cases on the cost continuum. They are good examples, though, of what American medical science can now do. Miracles happen every day and in many areas of care.

A few years ago, if a patient suffered from severe and persistent tremors, the result was often a lifetime of discomfort, embarrassment, and even pain. More recently, these patients could use powerful but inconsistently effective drugs that affected brain and body function in many ways while achieving only limited relief from the tremors.

Now, thanks to technology, care has improved for many of those patients. Today, a skilled surgeon can implant a tiny device called an Activa into the deep brain, turn on a switch, and, wonder of wonders, tremors cease.

Life for those patients immediately becomes much better. It's a miracle. It costs more than $17,000 for the device and approximately $25,000 more for the surgeon and hospital. Battery replacement for the device is required every three to five years for approximately $7,000. Other care costs are ongoing.[2]

That's a set of expenses that didn't exist five years ago. Health care premiums charged five years ago didn't have to collect any money to pay for neurostimulator devices, so health care premiums five years ago were lower.

How should we as Americans think about that particular care situation? If we believe that we each live only once and quality of life is important, is it worth the extra cost to have that amazing device implanted? Or should we as a society condemn that patient to a lifetime of tremors so we can save the money and keep insurance premium costs down?

Obviously, we will do the implants. When something works, we Americans use it—and pay the price. We perform miracles, and we expect them to be covered by our insurer.

The list of miracles goes on and on. Exciting new gamma knife therapy can target and destroy small tumors in the brain using highly focused gamma rays. The equipment costs $3.4 to $5 million to install. The treatment, done in either an outpatient or inpatient setting, costs $20,000 to $90,000 per procedure.[3] It's incredible technology. For some patients, it's the difference between life and death.

Lung volume reduction is used as a palliative surgical treatment for late-stage emphysema, enabling the patient to ventilate the remaining lung tissue more effectively. Hospital charges for this surgery range from $30,000 to $55,000.[4]

Transplants of bone marrow from another person for cancer treatment cost about $200,000 each.[5] People are alive today because of that treatment. But many of those survivors will have cancer relapse in a few years, triggering another round of miraculous care and significant expenses.

Islet cell transplantation for the treatment of diabetes helps the patient produce insulin and may reduce or eliminate the need for insulin shots. The procedure costs nearly $150,000.[6]

People whose hips fail get new hips inserted. New knees are becoming a commonplace surgery. Prosthetic ankles have allowed people whose lower limbs were lost to become joggers, even competitive runners.

These are all miracles. And they are all expensive.

700,000 Heart Stents a Year

New devices are developed all the time. If they work, they are used. That's the American way. Coronary artery stents, for example, are now being inserted into 700,000 hearts each year.[7] Vice President Dick Cheney was a highly publicized stent patient.

The stents are tiny tubes made of webbing. Their job is to keep vessels open and blood flowing in order to delay or avoid second heart attacks. Is that a good goal? Ask anyone who has had a first heart attack. Of course, it's a good goal. No one wants a second heart attack.

However, from 15 to 20 percent of these initial stents fail within six months because the stent gets clogged with scar tissue. These patients then must undergo further major treatment.[8] That clogging is a serious short-term setback. We really don't know at this point if there are any long-term setbacks. Because the procedures are relatively new, no one knows how many of those 700,000 stents will need surgical removal in ten years or twenty. The newest version of the stents is chemically coated. They seem to work twice as well.[9] They may also cost more than twice as much. And we also don't know how many of them will need to be pulled out and redone at some point in the future.

For now, however, putting all of those stents in people's chests seems like a very good risk to take. Why? Because second heart attacks are being measurably delayed for a high percentage of people.

The intent of the device is wonderful, and the immediate return is good 80 to 90 percent of the time. They achieve a miracle: an extension of life (an extension that, not incidentally, creates additional care expenses for the overall system).

Each of those stents, of course, costs money. The total market just for stents is now nearly $2 billion per year.[10] That's another new expense. Five years ago, stents were quite rare. Ten years ago, they didn't exist. Now they help millions of people stay alive.

So does the ventricular assist device, or heart pump, a device that helps patients with failing hearts maintain blood flow until the patient is ready for a heart transplant.

If the authors of this book personally had the need for a heart transplant, we'd definitely consider one of those pumps. The cost per pump per patient is roughly $75,000, nearly half the current cost of a full heart transplant. The introduction to the health care technology market of one new device, in other words, added 50 percent to the current cost of a heart transplant. It also slightly increased the number of transplants being done, because it keeps more people alive until a matching donor heart is available. That is yet another miracle that adds to the cumulative community cost of care.

Heart transplants themselves are a particularly good example of how technology and medical science constantly improve. Transplants were once an exotic, last-ditch, often unsuccessful, and always extremely expensive attempt to, at best, very briefly prolong lives. They were relatively rare. Today transplants are a common medical procedure and successful far more often than not when the right match is found between a patient and a donor heart. Patients survive for years, sometimes decades.

The transplants now cost anywhere from $150,000 to $500,000 per patient. Again, as with the tiny premature babies and the dialysis patients, that up-front cost gives us an expanded capability to keep people with failed hearts alive a lot longer so they can receive even more care. Transplant patients can live for a very long time. The post-transplant follow-up care—including ongoing antirejection drugs, anti-infection drugs, and biopsies to monitor for graft rejection—now runs roughly from $14,000 to $95,000 per year for the rest of that patient's life.

That ongoing cost is significant and far exceeds the actual individual health insurance premium paid each month by the average heart transplant patient. But when you look at the overall costs of the procedure and realize that people are benefiting immensely—living for many additional years and leading relatively normal, comparatively pain-free lives after the transplant—then it's pretty hard to argue that we as a society should save money by not doing that procedure and simply letting those people die.

The Six Million Dollar Man

If you start at the top of the head and move down the body, we can now insert enough prosthetic devices (knees, hips, ankles) and transplanted organs (hearts, lungs, kidneys, corneas) to create a six million dollar man or woman. It's hard to find a body part that can't be reconfigured, significantly repaired, or replaced. In almost all instances, the result is a better quality of life for the recipient of those prosthetics or procedures.

Miracles come in chemical versions as well as mechanical. We now have an array of amazing new drugs that make real differences in people's lives. The new drugs generally cost a lot more money than the drugs they replace.

Zofran, for example, is a wonder drug that helps prevent the nausea and vomiting associated with cancer chemotherapy. It costs $56.00 per day, replacing a less efficient drug that cost $3.25 per day.[11]

For people undergoing the miseries of cancer treatment, the reduction in suffering is another miracle, a fifty dollar per day miracle.

New antipsychotic agents such as Zyprexa and Risperdal are replacing older drugs that are generically available. The new drugs are more than ten times the daily cost of the old generics. Why are the new drugs used? Because, for some patients, they work better.

Until relatively recently, severe depression was not treated very effectively by drugs. Today we use a wonderful new class of antidepressants known as selective serotonin reuptake inhibitors (SSRIs). SSRI use has exploded. These drugs are now used by so many people that they frequently are a health plan's top cost in terms of total drug expenditures. These antidepressants, such as Prozac and Zoloft, have replaced generic drugs such as Elavil at approximately ten times the daily cost ($.25 per day compared to $2.64 per day).[12] Prozac and Zoloft are also given to millions of additional people who never would have received Elavil.

Deep vein thrombosis (DVT) can lead to pulmonary embolism. In the past, patients with DVT, or at high risk for DVT, were hospitalized to receive intravenous therapy. Now a drug, Lovenox, given subcutaneously can be used in an outpatient setting. The cost of Lovenox is about $40 to $75 per day.[13]

Looking ahead, we can see a huge potential drug cost looming for new antibiotic drugs. Overuse of the less expensive antibiotic drugs has resulted in several frightening strains of bacteria that are now drug resistant. People are suffering greatly and even dying from some of the staphylococcus strains that eat their flesh. Those germs laugh at the old pharmaceuticals that used to fight them off. Entertainer Rosie O'Donnell's battle with staphylococcus was well publicized.

Even the current drugs of last resort, like vancomycin, are not working consistently against the new diseases. At one point, we could stop those diseases with ampicillin at $0.39 per dose. Then we had to fall back on cefazolin at $0.90 per dose. Now we need to use linezolid (Zyvox) at $58.10 per dose—and even it doesn't always work.[14]

The drug costs are just a fraction of the total care cost for patients who are attacked by these new disease strains. These antibiotic-resistant staph patients can easily run up hospital bills in the tens of thousands of dollars before discharge. Bills for some patients exceed $100,000. Some patients die. Many are crippled for life or seriously disfigured.

New drugs are under development. Some may work. None will be cheap.

The drugs that used to kill off tuberculosis and staphylococcus easily and inexpensively are all now useless against some of the newer and more virulent strains of those bacteria. The new drugs cost thousands of dollars and work inconsistently at best. If infections caused by staphylococcus and tuberculosis ever become rampant in this country, we will see another cost explosion, one with far fewer miracles and many truly tragic outcomes. Likewise, if diseases like the West Nile virus become common in our country, our approach to care will create increased costs for the entire economy. In the rest of the world, most of these patients die because effective, proven therapy is unavailable. In the United States, heroic, high-intensity, and high-cost care will be the order of the day in response to epidemics.

But those are next year's problems. For now, we're primarily paying for today's miracles. Today's miracles work. We are constantly seeing major improvements in just about every area of care. It's all extremely encouraging if you are a patient.

Surgical techniques have also gotten better. Lasers have replaced scalpels for hernia repair and removing skin cancer. Gallbladder removal used to require opening up the abdomen for major surgery. That surgery can now be done laparoscopically, through a very small incision using a miniature camera. The new procedure involves fewer risks or complications. It also speeds recovery by four weeks, sometimes resulting in real savings to employers for less time lost from work.

That particular new procedure costs only slightly more per patient than the old. That's not the major cost driver. The cost issue is volume. Because the new approach is less invasive and works so well, many more people, especially the elderly, now undergo this procedure. That ease of use has, for example, significantly increased the total cost of gallbladder surgery in this country.[15]

Is that good care? Yes—for people who need gallbladder removal. It's another medical miracle and, like most other medical miracles, it costs money. Every insurance company is paying an additional price for that care.

The list of expense increases goes on and on. Today we are facing a shortage of a crucial medical product: blood. Thirteen million units of blood were used in 2000, and demand is increasing at 6 to 8 percent while donations are up by just 2 to 3 percent.

Again, technology is coming to the rescue. Soon we may have the option of using artificial blood, which would have a much longer shelf life and would eliminate the need for matching blood types. That would be another medical miracle. But the cost impact of this new product is also probably going to be high. The average unit of donated blood now costs about $130. Prices for artificial blood are estimated to be anywhere from $300 to $1,000 per unit. Don't bet on $300.[16]

If It Works, We Use It

Think of the whole process this way: every time a wonderful new procedure is proven to work, it gets used. If it works, it is paid for by our insurance process. We each then share in the costs of the procedure through our premium. Care is continuously better because the money to pay for that care is now readily available. The pooling process and insurance premium increases let us all work together to make that money and care available.

The question is, Are all of those medical technology improvements worth the cost?

None of us would want to return to the health care tool kit of only a decade ago. New implants, new procedures, new drugs, and new imaging technologies help doctors diagnose more accurately and treat more effectively. Earlier intervention in the lives of people with chronic conditions can help prolong lives and reduce discomfort and pain. Almost all of the innovations improve care. That's indisputably good.

Some of the new procedures actually don't work. A recent study showed that the most common arthroscopic surgery done on knees had no more impact than a placebo surgery done on knees with comparable problems.[17] More than 80,000 of those surgeries were done last year, which may well have been wasted money for everyone involved. (The whole issue of valid, science-based care is discussed later in this book.)

The point to keep in mind here is that most of the new drugs and procedures add real value to people's lives. We need to recognize as a society, however, that just about every one of those innovations is expensive. We use all of them because that is the way the system is set up in this country today. Once we use them, we have to pay for them. (In some cases we probably pay too much, a topic explored in a later chapter.)

Looming just ahead of us is a highly likely explosion of costs that will result from the new genetic sciences. We may soon be able to tailor drugs, treatments, and even gene transplants that are specific to individuals with both dire and chronic diseases. The curative potential for those treatments is huge. The potential costs are even higher. It's possible to imagine a doubling of total treatments costs from that one area of science alone.

We are just seeing the beginning of that trend. We have some serious decisions to make as a society about the overall cost of care and our expectations about the maximum use of care that will need to guide us all as that whole new world of genetic science reaches full bloom. Those miracles could make today's miracles look relatively unimpressive, and cheap.

But that's for tomorrow.

For now, one key fact to consider is that medical miracles happen every day in this country, every minute, in fact. They all cost money. Another key fact to consider is that American health care, good as it is when we are really sick, leaves a lot to be desired when it comes to consistency, safety, and giving us all the value we pay for.

So how inconsistent and unsafe is U.S. health care? You might be surprised.

. . . .

Unsafe at Any Cost

Maybe the single most amazing thing about American health care today is how inconsistent, unfocused, and even dangerous that care can be.

Between 44,000 and 98,000 Americans die each year in hospital accidents.[1] That may be a conservative estimate. That number doesn't include near misses and nonfatal accidents. Those numbers are far higher. Your likelihood of being injured by negligence during a hospital stay is nearly 40 percent greater than the likelihood of an airline's mishandling your luggage.[2]

How does that accidental death rate compare to other activities? Your chance of dying from simply being in a hospital (not due to the illness that put you there) is four hundred times more likely than your risk of death from traveling by train, forty times higher than driving a car, and twenty times higher than flying in a commercial aircraft.[3]

The hospital accident numbers are sobering. They speak urgently to the need to be much more systematic about our care. Airlines do a good job on safety because they focus directly and explicitly on safety issues. Pilots are taught teamwork. More important, airlines do systematic analyses of every accident and every near miss. These analyses are continuously translated into specific systematic changes designed to prevent future reoccurrences of the dangerous event.

Consequently, notwithstanding the terrible events of September 11, 2001, air travel is extremely safe—much safer than hospital admissions. The chance of dying in a domestic jet accident is approximately one in 8 million.[4] Only a few planes crash every year. By contrast, accidents in U.S. hospitals kill the equivalent of a 747 full of patients every twenty-four hours.

In many settings, hospitals avoid conducting airline-like studies of near misses because of the threat of lawsuits and financial liability. The same types of studies and incident reporting processes that make airplane travel safe can be done only at significant legal risk to the hospitals that should be undergoing similar activities. Many hospitals, to avoid liability, avoid doing those studies with very much enthusiasm or vigor. That isn't good for any of us.

These frightening statistics about hospital safety come from a safety report, "To Err Is Human," published by the Institute of Medicine (IOM) in 1999. Since the IOM wrote its sobering report, we've learned quite a lot more about the nature of hospital-based patient accidents. We now know that hundreds of wrong-site surgeries occur every year in this country. Here are some typical incidents as reported in the *New York Times:* two doctors accused of operating on the wrong side of a patient's brain; one doctor who did surgery on the wrong section of a spinal cord; another doctor removing the left kidney of a seventy-nine-year-old man who had cancer in his right kidney; and another doctor operating on a healthy knee, rather than an injured one—the second such mistake for that particular doctor in five years. The *New York Times* article also pointed out that wrong-site surgery is rarely the fault of a single person but is generally caused by flaws in the hospital's operating procedures and the lack of systematic safety procedures to prevent these mistakes.[5]

In a recent study of wrong-site surgery cases, the Joint Commission on Accreditation of Healthcare Organizations cited several factors contributing to errors: the involvement of multiple surgeons, performance of several different procedures during one surgery, and pressure from hospital administrators to finish surgery quickly. A systematic response to each of those factors is both possible and desirable.[6]

Dr. Don Berwick, of Harvard Medical School and president of the Institute for Healthcare Improvement, believes that "the remedy is not to say, 'who did it . . .' but rather, 'how has our system led to such dire consequences, and how can we make the system so robust that we can account for predictable human frailty?'"[7]

Cut at the X; No, Don't Cut at the X

The need for systematic solutions is evident. In one Minnesota community, providers looking at the issue of hospital safety discovered that one local hospital asked the surgeons doing a procedure to put an X on the arm that was *not* to be operated on. A nearby hospital, also trying to be safe, required surgeons to mark the body part (for example, arm, breast, leg) that *was* to be operated on. Many surgeons practiced at both hospitals and so had to remember where they were to know what each marker meant. Those hospitals are now using the same system as a first step toward reducing those kinds of unnecessary systems-created safety problems.[8]

Hospital Safety Issues Are Just the Tip of the Iceberg

Hospital safety issues have been widely publicized and don't need a lot of attention here. What has been much less widely publicized have been the much greater safety issues that exist in nonhospital settings across the entire health care system. The most dangerous and alarming issues actually have nothing to do with hospitals or hospital accidents. They have to do with inconsistent and dysfunctional clinical patterns of care.

Millions of people die, are maimed, or are placed in jeopardy of being damaged every year across this country because our overall care system is inconsistent, nonsystematic, and even idiosyncratic in the delivery of care. Dr. John Wennberg's studies on the wide variations in care patterns across the country offer sobering proof of how much danger and inconsistency exist in U.S. health care.[9]

Inappropriate Heart Care Is Unsafe
and Expensive Heart Care

There are, sadly, many, many areas where inappropriate care causes
huge costs in dollars, suffering, and deaths. Follow-up clinical care
for a heart attack is one example. Inappropriate follow-up care for
heart attacks causes literally hundreds of thousands of people to die
prematurely. Inappropriate follow-up care is far more common than
anyone wants to admit. A second IOM study, *Crossing the Quality
Chasm*, dealt very specifically with that issue.[10] For the most part,
both the public and the news media ignored that second IOM study.
The topics of clinical safety were apparently too complex for quick
absorption. The facts, however, are sobering. The care system puts
patients at risk every day, invisibly.

If a diabetic were told that a particular brand of coffee would increase his or her chance of going blind or losing a limb by 60 percent, the person would likely react with a high level of energy,
refusing the coffee and avoiding that risk. But for most diabetics,
patterns of clinical care that create that same high level of risk
occur every day, and America's diabetics have no clue that the danger even exists. That's unsafe care.

Solid medical science tells us that when a patient has a heart attack, the likelihood of that person's dying from a second heart
attack can be reduced by over 40 percent by administering beta
blockers to the patient.

No one disputes the science. The treatment saves lives. But
nearly 40 percent of American patients do not receive that necessary care. Nearly 40 percent do not receive beta blockers. If you add
up all of the heart attack victims in the country and assume a 40
percent noncompliance rate by American physicians, then that puts
440,000 Americans at a significantly higher risk of death every single day.[11] And no one in this country even keeps track of who that
40 percent are. Outside of some health maintenance organization–
related quality tracking systems, there is no program in this coun-

try for systematically measuring and reporting the actual outcomes of any care. We simply expect millions of independent, often over-worked caregivers to all somehow "do it right."

That blind trust approach is not good enough. It doesn't create safe care for all patients. Because of the inconsistencies in the way American caregivers approach care, nearly half of the people who have heart attacks are left at high risk of having multiple attacks and dying.

That is a safety issue, a personal safety issue for those patients. And it is a cost issue. Those unnecessary heart attacks are driving up the cost of care.

Medical Inconsistency Creates Unsafe Care for Congestive Heart Failure Patients

Congestive heart failure (CHF) has an even more dramatic level of variation in patient safety. Congestive heart failure patients who go into crisis are at very high risk of dying. Those crises are life threatening and absolutely terrifying. People drown in their own body fluids.

Most of those terrible CHF crises don't have to happen. Most patients who go through that medical hell do so unnecessarily. Therefore, care for those patients is, by those standards, unsafe.

In contrast, informed caregivers, including those at HealthPartners, who use current medical best practices and systematic team-based care for CHF patients can reduce these life-threatening crises by more than 60 percent.[12] Kaiser Permanente of Ohio has reduced CHF death rates to less than half of the state average.

Both HealthPartners and Kaiser Permanente have made major commitments to providing consistent, science-based care to their members—and both have had major successes with conditions like CHF.

But less than 10 percent of the CHF patient population in this country gets that needed care. The other 90 percent are still getting unsafe care, which significantly increases the likelihood that they will suffer unnecessarily and die too soon.

Do the patients know which doctors deliver what level of care? Absolutely not. A small amount of quality data is available at some macrolevels for some auditors, and a limited number of large multi-specialty medical groups perform their own internal quality screens and activities, but for the most part, no one in our current non-system of care either records care outcomes or uses them to improve care.

Even more troubling than the lack of information for patients is the lack of processes to ensure the best quality. There is also no systematic process, similar to airline quality improvement practices, that brings all doctors up to speed on the new best treatments for CHF patients. As a result, a lot of people die prematurely, and others suffer unnecessary trauma.

The cost in human lives is unacceptable. The cost in dollars is also huge. It costs a lot more to do CHF care wrong. It saves a lot of money to do it right.

Unsafe Diabetes, Flu, and Prenatal Care

The same patterns of inconsistent and unsafe care exist for many other conditions. Fewer than half of the doctors in the United States provide full and appropriate follow-up care to their patients with diabetes, for example. That is a huge problem for Americans with diabetes.

Diabetes is the number one cause of blindness, amputation, and kidney failure in this country. Most people in kidney dialysis units are there because of their diabetes. The risk of stroke is 2.5 times higher for people with diabetes.[13] Diabetes substantially increases the risk of death in heart patients. It's a disease whose patients now consume nearly 25 percent of the money spent by Medicare. There has been a 33 percent increase in the number of people with diabetes in this country since 1990.[14] The sharpest rise—a 70 percent increase—was among people in their thirties.[15]

Again, the sad (but invisible) truth is that the current system of care in this country is unsafe for most diabetics. Medical research has shown that when doctors provide appropriate care and help patients manage blood sugar levels and when doctors detect and treat complications at very early stages, patients are 40 percent less likely to incur the terrible crippling or fatal complications of that disease.[16] Patients don't know these important facts. They rely on their physicians and other caregivers to create medical safety, and the system lets them down. Dialysis units are full of patients with failing kidneys who would not be there if the patients had received safe care.

Similar patterns exist for people at high risk of death from the flu. Proactive programs can cut those deaths due to flu complications by 50 percent.[17] People without those systematic programs are 50 percent less safe.

Similarly, systematic, carefully implemented preterm birth programs can cut premature deliveries by half, clearly a safety issue for each baby. When babies are born very prematurely, many die. If they live, they can end up with a lifetime of medical misery. So it is particularly important to know that careful and systematic screening, timely and well-organized interventions, and maternal education and behavior changes can cut preterm births by more than half.

Barely Half of the Patients Received Best Care

Hospitals are taking the heaviest publicity hits these days for patient safety. That's really not at all fair when heart patients, diabetics, pregnant women and infants, asthmatics, and dozens of other categories of young and old patients also find themselves far too vulnerable to the worst consequences of their diseases because of inconsistent, unsafe, and unsystematic care.

A major study to be released later in 2003 looked at 18,000 patient physician charts in communities across the country. Care delivered to those patients was compared to up-to-date best practice protocols agreed to by some of the best medical minds in the country. How well did the American care system do? Not well at all. Only 55 percent of the patients received their care in keeping with the current best practices.[18]

In cases where the medical science was particularly clear and strongly supported by "level one" (the very best) evidence, the number rose to only 57 percent. (In evaluating the validity of medical research, three categories of evidence are used. Level one means that there are multiple, reaffirming, clinically valid studies that reach a common conclusion.) Fifty-seven percent is not a very impressive or reassuring level of performance. According to that same major study, 68,000 Americans die unnecessarily each year just due to poorly treated hypertension alone. That hypertension death rate, all by itself, equals the highly publicized death rate from hospital accidents. Another 10,000 patients died because of inadequately treated pneumonia. The researchers looked at two dozen medical conditions and found similar results for every single one. That isn't good news for American patients. Or payers.

That is, for sure, not "safe" care.

Unsafe Care Is Also Unnecessarily Expensive Care

The issue of medical consistency is first and foremost a patient safety issue. It is, however, also a significant—even major—cost issue. The good news is that it generally costs less to do care right than it does to do it wrong.

The net financial cost of those inconsistencies is immense. A study done by the Midwestern Business Group on Health estimated that 30 percent of all health care dollars were spent on inappropriate care.[19] The cost in human suffering has to be added to the cost in dollars if that is, in fact, an accurate estimate. We know for a fact that hospital accidents, which too often result in patients' acquiring infections, create high bills. So do inappropriate dosages of prescription drugs or even drugs that are given to patients entirely in error. Those costs add billions of dollars to the U.S. health care cost structure.

Unnecessary and avoidable episodes of congestive heart failure crisis also adds billions of dollars in unnecessary expenses.

Unnecessary and avoidable preterm births easily add many more hundreds of millions of dollars in completely wasteful expenses. The fact that people with diabetes now use nearly 25 percent of all Medicare dollars speaks for itself. That number would be much lower if all of those with diabetes received best care.

As we noted in Chapter One, the good news is that after the fact—after the harm is done—we can perform medical miracles, though often at huge expense, to keep those harmed patients alive longer. A much better solution would be to prevent millions of people from being so badly harmed in the first place.

There is some irony in our willingness to spend huge amounts of money to repair damage that should have been prevented by the care system. A cynic might note that the typical fee-for-service American payment approach generates huge fees for medical procedures, huge fees for hospital treatments, and no fees for preventing either the situations or the health problems that necessitate those expensive treatments. The problem may not be that we over-reward treatment, but that we significantly underpay for prevention and for managing outcomes.

Right now, our increasing competence in keeping care system–harmed people alive is a significant cost escalator. We need an equivalent decrease in the number of people being harmed. We need two strategies: one to treat those harmed patients and one to keep the patients from being harmed in the first place. We need to keep those harmed people alive, but we also need to put as much or more energy into preventing the complications and crisis in the first place.

The Best Care Systems Really Do Improve Care

This isn't a pipe dream. It can be done. For diabetes, for example, systematic application of medical best practices can have a major positive impact on care. The very best medical teams have proved that diabetes complications can be significantly reduced. Some of that information is actually available to the public. Look for health plan comparative quality report scores on diabetic care to get a sense of what can be done. (The HEDIS® studies by the National Committee for Quality Assurance [NCQA] contain that information. HEDIS, which stands for Health Plan Employer Data and Information Set, is a set of performance measures that tell how well health plans perform in key areas. Health plans must collect data in a standardized way so that comparisons are fair and valid. HEDIS results are posted on the NCQA.org Web site.)

Many of the best care systems either set up their own science-based diabetes care protocols or follow the care standards set by the American Diabetes Association (ADA). Systematic approaches work. The best care systems do twice as well as the worst systems in taking care of people with diabetes. The ADA and NCQA know which providers do well and which do poorly. So should the patients.

Sadly, the news media have not been interested in that story. They have not been able to grasp the incredible value of the new ADA and NCQA medical provider evaluation system so the public doesn't know which care systems and medical groups do well.

A number of health plans and medical groups, including Health-Partners and Kaiser Permanente, have invested time, energy, and resources in creating evidence-based best care protocols for a wide range of diseases. The results of pilot programs on various sites have been overwhelmingly positive. At HealthPartners, physicians and care teams have cut episodes of congestive heart failure crisis by over 60 percent and flu deaths by 50 percent. They have put systematic programs in place to reduce preterm births to less than half of the national average. HealthPartners physicians have put programs in place to reduce asthma crisis by over half. They have

---

HEDIS® is a registered trademark of the National Committee for Quality Assurance (NCQA).

achieved a 98 percent success rate on the appropriate use of beta blockers after heart attack compared to a national average of less than 60 percent.

By doing a careful analysis of the accuracy rate of radiologists reading mammograms, Kaiser Permanente has pilot programs in place that have identified a significant variation in physician skill levels. The resultant retraining and correction process made a major improvement in early cancer detection levels, reducing the number of cancers detected later than Stage One from 14 percent to fewer than 10 percent. That systematic review of physician performance has already saved lives. It points the way to a new level of accountability for delivering and improving care. In other less organized settings, those kinds of reviews simply are not done.

Systems like these have proven beyond any doubt that safer care is practical and possible. It takes systematic thinking about care and then strategic planning and programs to improve care. It takes enlightened physician leaders who know how to apply systems thinking to care. These systems save millions of dollars a year through these programs and also save lives. The benefits to patients are priceless.

Every doctor wants to do the right thing. There aren't any physicians who knowingly provide inadequate care. But there are now approximately 23,000 medical journals published each year.[20] No one can keep up. No single physician can be entirely current. Professional studies have shown that it can take fifteen to twenty years for doctors and hospitals to incorporate new scientific evidence about drugs and devices into their practices.[21]

Inconsistency Happens; Consistency Can Be Created

The book *Strong Medicine*, written by one of us (George Halvorson), looked at 135 doctors who were asked how they would treat a particular condition for a particular patient. They came up with eighty-two separate treatments.[22] Why? Because some physicians graduated from medical school last month. Others graduated a year ago, or twenty years ago, or forty years ago. Some attended seminars on the topic. Others read articles on the topic. Some articles were recent. Some weren't. Some physicians were influenced by drug sales representatives. Each drug company, of course, has its own perspective about which drugs should be prescribed, a perspective that doesn't necessarily coincide with objective studies showing which drugs actually do the best job.

So inconsistency happens. That's understandable, particularly when so many American doctors still function as solo practitioners or with a single partner. These doctors are trying to run a business, see a full load of patients, hire and fire staff, comply with all employment laws and tax codes, and then do all necessary medical reading and learning, in addition to all of the other professional, political, and personal time pressures that make life today so challenging. It isn't easy. Those doctors need help to stay current—help that needs to be extended to the physician right at the point when patients are receiving care.

The model we advocate is explained more fully in Chapter Twelve. It is a systematic approach that creates review teams of the brightest and best physicians and other caregivers. Those teams study a given condition. They constantly review the most current information about diagnosis and treatment. Then they build and continuously update evidence-based care guidelines based on the most current science and data. Their findings are then communicated on an ongoing basis to all of the other doctors in the medical group or caregiver network. That approach seems simple and logical. In the real world of care, it's revolutionary. The not-yet-published results showing that only 55 percent of doctors complied with best care practices makes the case for systematic care improvement beyond dispute.

The seminal work done by Dr. John Wennberg on regional care variation makes that same point very well. It is clear beyond any doubt that there are huge variations in care patterns, region to region, and that care in some areas of the country is more dangerous and wasteful than care in other areas. That variation creates problems for patients that simply should not exist. We need best care, not idiosyncratic care. Wennberg's studies also showed that the costs of care could also be reduced by upwards of 20 percent simply by having all doctors rise to the level of the most effective doctors. That doesn't seem as if it should be an insurmountable goal.

We believe that the best doctors should and must be the leaders in identifying best care.

Doctors Must Lead the Process

The authors of this book work for health plans closely aligned with particular multispecialty medical practices. Our role in that closely linked model is to both encourage and reward the development of solid, physician-led care protocol processes. It is also to help distribute the physician-developed guidelines (along with the science that underpins them) and to accept those guideline as the preferred mode of care.

It's important to do this process right. We do not believe in rules for physicians. Rules don't work. Medicine changes too fast to impose rules. Individual patients can have complications that invalidate rules.

Rules-based medicine, we believe, is wrong. But guidelines-based medicine is clearly superior to the kind of fiercely nonsystematic idiosyncratic approach that creates eighty-two different treatments for just one patient.

The IOM report on care quality, *Crossing the Quality Chasm*, identifies clearly the problems and inconsistencies that exist in American health care today. The authors describe a better system— one that uses science-based care protocols as the foundation for best care. We agree entirely and strongly recommend that report to anyone wanting to improve health care quality in America today.

An Automated Medical Record Is the Critical Next Step

To fully realize the benefits of medical best practices at a patient-specific level, it's time to make a huge improvement in the physician's tool kit. We need to bring medical information availability into the twenty-first century—bringing the use of computer technology into the exam room. Right now, almost all physicians need to rely on their own memory for large portions of their treatment information. They also are forced to rely on paper medical records that leave a lot to be desired. Instead of having splintered medical records in paper files in multiple sites, doctors need a single patient-focused consolidated medical record that is constantly available in the exam room at the exact point and time of care. That computer system needs to have in it not only all information about each patient, but also all information about the patient's disease and the best possible treatments for that disease.

As medical science progresses exponentially, it is unfair to both physicians and patients to expect the physician's memory to be sufficient to keep all care practices and patient follow-up steps current and up to speed.

That automated system also needs to meet all confidentiality standards while providing each patient with data, information, and useful behavioral support. It's time for medicine to move beyond the obsolete human memory–based exam room interactions of the 1900s to take full advantage of the best technology of the new millennium. The best pathway to safe and consistent care, we believe, will be electronic, giving physicians the necessary tools and then making those tools easy to use.

It's hard to imagine how difficult it is to deliver consistent, top-quality care without a tool of that nature. Every other profession has managed to incorporate the computer to improve the way that the practitioners do their work. Architects, engineers, and lawyers all use the computer to supplement their brains. It's time for medicine to follow that same path.

This is a great opportunity. The current approach is badly flawed.

In most medical care settings, physicians have no systems in place to remind them of what best care is for any given condition. Physicians are expected to remember hundreds of treatment patterns and to remember which patients need what follow-up care. The only work tool that most doctors have to help ensure consistent delivery of best care is an old-fashioned, badly organized paper medical record—often hard to read, too often unavailable at the point of care, and generally containing only incomplete pieces of patient history, with no specific next steps for patient care.

To make matters even worse, each doctor site now generally maintains a separate physically isolated medical record, so if a patient is receiving care from multiple physicians at multiple sites, no doctor at any site is ever fully aware of what is being done at each of the other sites. The current epidemic of dangerous drug interactions results in part from Doctor A's having no way of knowing what drug Doctor B has prescribed. The current lack of follow-up care for chronic diseases is also caused in part by the inadequacies of that manual, paper-based record-keeping approach.

An automated medical record (AMR) not only cleans up that confusion, it also has the ability to remind the doctor in real time that particular tests need to be run or particular drugs need to be prescribed. The AMR can even tell the doctor if the patient actually filled the prior prescription. The benefits of an AMR are so overwhelmingly obvious that it is amazing that caregivers don't already have that tool at their disposal.

The next major improvement in U.S. health care will result from the carefully designed and consistent use of AMRs. But that process has just begun and is helping at very few sites. In the rest of the country, we have the embarrassing, unacceptable, and dangerous 55 percent compliance with best medical science as a direct consequence of not having computers used as physician tools at the point where the patients would benefit the most. When an automated record-keeping system exists, then the newest science can be made available to the doctor at the point of care delivery. And when the science changes, as it often does, those changes can also be communicated quickly and effectively through a computerized system rather than relying on a complex flow of journal articles and memos to get the attention of overworked care providers during their "free" hours. That ability to simply update medical science for practitioners is, all by itself, a major and overdue enhancement for care delivery.

Think about the alternative to that process. Most doctors have to seek out that information on their own. Even in those few settings where care protocols are updated regularly, the task of communicating each of these updates to all physicians can be immense—laborious and labor intensive. If two thousand doctors in a network have learned a protocol for simple cystitis, for example, through seminars, letters, professional journals, and collegial interaction, and then the science changes, it takes a huge effort to get the new information and science in front of all two thousand doctors. It's possible to do, but it takes a major effort and considerable time. And that's just for one condition. How can any nonelectronic system effectively update care science for dozens, even hundreds, of medical conditions? The science of medicine will be much more current when appropriate computerized communication tools are in place for all physicians. Without these tools, medicine has little or no hope of turning that embarrassing and unacceptable national 55 percent best practice score into a 99 percent best practice score. And care will continue to be unsafe for far too many patients.

Consumers Deserve to Know How Provider Performance Compares

Patients also ought to know how well different caregivers and caregiver teams do in creating outcomes. We started down that path at HealthPartners in Minnesota about four years ago and can testify that it's valuable to consumers who are making decisions about the providers they will use. HealthPartners uses the Internet, for example, to let patients with diabetes know how well local caregivers do in helping their own patients control blood sugar. They let patients know how well various local orthopedic surgeons do in creating satisfied patients after knee and hip surgery. Diabetic patients find that kind of information useful. People contemplating knee surgery find it invaluable and can make care decisions accordingly.

Informed patients can help create a care marketplace based on quality and value, not just market image and geographic proximity.

Care Improves When Quality Is Reported Publicly

We know from the Internet-based programs HealthPartners has run in Minnesota that measuring and reporting the outcomes of care also improve care system performance. As one example, the care team that had one of the lowest (worst) scores on diabetic care in the first year that HealthPartners measured relative diabetes performance became the highest-scoring care team after two years. These doctors had no idea of how badly they had been doing before the measurement process began. They had believed they were doing really well. They were good doctors who knew, in fact, exactly what do to, but their medical group had no systems in place to support the quality and type of care they wanted, so they failed.

They had a first-year 25 percent best practice score compared to a network-wide first-year average of 54 percent and a best practice score of 67 percent.[23] Once those low-scoring doctors learned how badly they had done, they were stunned. They studied the prior year's winners and copied them. They put systems in place, reinforced them with staff and patients, and climbed to a 75 percent score, one of the best around in a world that doesn't have an automated medical record to help the doctors get to even higher scores.

Progress can be made. All of the other care systems improved as well, of course. Patients across the community benefited.

We did not publicly report the first-year score for those particular low-scoring physicians because we knew they were good doctors.

Our goal is not to make anyone good look bad. Our goal is to improve care. So after showing them their low score, we told them, "A year from now, your scores will go on the Internet."

Although we believe those doctors may have made the improvements without the threat of publicity, the reporting process created a useful time frame in which to make improvements.

HealthPartners has used that two-step approach in other areas of care as well, including heart care: measuring quietly and using the data privately to improve care for a year or more before letting the public and the patients see comparative numbers. In heart care, for example, HealthPartners' current studies show a huge variation in patient satisfaction with cardiac care performance, ranging from an 83 percent very satisfied response level for some groups down to a 54 percent very satisfied response level from patients of other groups.[24] Within the groups are physicians with patient satisfaction ratings as low as 37 percent and as high as 100 percent.[25]

HealthPartners is reporting that particular set of caregiver-specific data to Minnesotans and working with each of these low-scoring groups to improve performance. HealthPartners will remeasure and publicly report on a periodic basis. Right now, a couple of the physician groups who were measured are in shock. Like the low-scoring diabetes team, they had no idea that they had so much room for improvement.

We believe in this performance measurement and reporting model because it works. It makes care safe for patients. On a measure like testing for diabetes blood sugar in control, HealthPartners has managed to hit scores of 79 percent. The national average is less than 63 percent.[26] The 79 percent figure places HealthPartners above the ninetieth percentile (in the top 10 percent of all health plans). This isn't an accident. It was earned, not just discovered. It helps keep patients safely away from kidney failure and other complications of diabetes.

Health plans tightly aligned with medical group practices are far from perfect and certainly don't make any claim to that effect. But in dozens of important areas of care, they have proven with pilot programs that huge improvements can be made when skilled and enlightened medical leadership uses systematic, science-based approaches to deliver and enhance care.

When you realize that most people in kidney dialysis units are there because diabetes caused their kidneys to fail, then the national average of only 36 percent of America's patients being examined for protein in the urine, a sign of kidney damage by diabetes, is pathetic.[27] It truly is unsafe care. Walk through a dialysis unit and ask the people hooked up to those blood treatment machines how they feel about having failed kidneys.

The human tragedies are immense. We can do much better.

There is tremendous resistance to this model. America's health care delivery system is in a state of denial about safety and consistent care issues. It also is in a state of denial about the value of using the computer in the exam room to ensure the doctor's ability to help patients and optimally treat disease. Some of the best multispecialty medical groups have gone down the path of automating both their medical records and treatment guidelines, but many have not. Without that tool, best practices are very hard to achieve, and significant levels of improvement are difficult to attain.

The Value of Intervention Isn't Widely Known

Because the public at large has no idea of how inconsistent care can be, the vast majority of patients surveyed say their strong personal preference would be for their doctors to be totally independent of any external influence relative to their pattern of care. That preference is understandable but unfortunate. The very best medical groups create strong and consistent internal standards of care. So do the best health plans. But outside of those settings, the situation leaves a lot to be desired.

Without those standards, what results is a 25 percent adequacy score on a comprehensive diabetic quality measure.[28] A lack of standards results in heart patients' dying prematurely because they had unnecessary second heart attacks. Not setting standards results in terrifying and totally unnecessary episodes of CHF crisis.

If the nonstandard approach to care prevails in this country, then costs will continue to explode, and we will continue to see two times too many congestive heart failure patients lying in hospital beds, gasping for air, drowning in their own fluids, and wondering if they are going to live until morning.

These standards and care protocols need to be set by physicians, not actuaries or managers. They need to be based on best care and patient outcomes. They also need to be set in a way that gives the public peace of mind about the quality and accountability of care.

We Need a Focus on the Real Quality Issues

Improving the safety and consistency of care in all care sites is an issue where open public dialogue is essential. That dialogue will not happen as long as the press ignores statistical quality reports and instead politicizes a subset of photogenic, anecdote-based quality issues. We need a public discussion based on science and data, not incidents and rhetoric. We need an informed community discussion on patient safety, with the real issues put on the table for everyone to discuss and debate. We also need the purchasers of care to support that whole safety agenda and to strongly encourage the use of automated medical records with care protocol reminders embedded in them.

Why Isn't Quality a Market Driver Today?

A key question that might be asked at this point is why the American public tolerates an extremely expensive care delivery nonsystem that provides best care only 55 percent of the time. Why, you might ask, haven't market forces emerged to take advantage of that situation?

There are a couple of reasons that quality has not become a true market differentiation factor between health plans and care providers. One is that most Americans don't realize how inconsistent or even dangerous care can be. It's hard for anyone to appreciate a solution to any problem until people first appreciate, or at least become aware of, the actual problem. Most Americans are in a state of blissful ignorance relative to the care delivery risks they are facing, so people in general aren't looking for those risks to be reduced.

Second, even if they've heard that care delivery is inconsistent, the vast majority of consumers believe that their own personal physician is in the 55 percent category (caregivers prescribing adequate care), not the 45 percent category (caregivers who are not). People have no way of knowing which providers are which for any given type of care because there are no data available to help figure out which caregivers are doing well and which leave a lot to be desired.

That situation is compounded a bit by the fact that both caregivers and health plans have done a relatively bad job of selling quality in any persuasive or effective way. It is "politically incorrect" and "impolite" inside American health care to point out the disparities in both care outcomes and care practices. Plans are afraid of making doctors angry if the topic is raised. Physicians tend not to point out the performance problems of other physicians. The current macrosystem is not set up to either self-report or self-correct.

So the Wennberg data sets are all ignored by the various caregivers and plans. The news media do not spend much time on these stories either, so it's perfectly understandable that patients are not demanding quality information as part of the caregiver or health plan selection process.

All of these issues are exacerbated by the fact that the science of recording and reporting quality is in its early stages. The quality reporting mechanisms improve every year, but they haven't been particularly useful until very recently for consumers.

Even now, the NCQA data that are available about overall health plan networks can be very compelling at aggregate levels, but are not very useful at the individual caregiver level, where consumers make real choices. All of that needs to change if we are going to make quality an effective component in the health care marketplace. Thanks to the IOM and organizations like the Institute for Healthcare Improvement, the current trends of unsafe and inconsistent care are finally visible. The question is how to turn that information into data that improve both care delivery and consumer decision making. Systems like that of HealthPartners and Kaiser Permanente have proved that better approaches and better outcomes are possible. Adding automated medical record systems to the mix creates a much needed possibility and potentiality for truly superb and very safe care. It also creates a whole new level of access to data that will have real market reform potential. Patient safety needs to be a top priority for us all. As we make the quality of care better and safety levels higher, patients will benefit and costs will go down.

For now, however, care is inconsistent and costs are increasing. So who is really paying for all of that care?

3

. . . .

Who Really Pays for
All of That Care?

Medical miracles feel free to most Americans. Why? Because typical insurance coverage in this country is so complete that most people who have heart transplants, for example, pay only a few hundred dollars in incidental copayments as their total out-of-pocket expense for a medical procedure that costs a quarter of a million dollars. That feels free.

Of course, money, lots of money, actually changes hands when these procedures are performed. Surgeons collect fees. Hospitals get paid their charges. Nurses receive salaries. Most patients, however, are very effectively insulated from each of those major incident-based costs of care by their insurance coverage. The cost of that coverage has been borne primarily by people's employers or, in the case of Medicare and Medicaid patients, by the government. Certainly, costs have been incurred, but the whole process is almost invisible to the actual patient.

Health care is a unique sector of our economy. In most other sectors, people pay directly for a service when the service is rendered. Food is purchased by the piece or pound. You dine in a restaurant, you pay the bill; your car is repaired, you pay for the parts and labor. By paying directly out of pocket, the consumer has a clear sense of the cost and the value of each service or product used. Health care is entirely different. An extremely expensive and a very cheap medical procedure are equally cost free to most patients. Insurance blurs the cost and value of care perception for most individuals.

In fact, Americans are so used to being insulated from the costs of health care that many become extremely upset when insurance doesn't cover some level of care. If, for example, an insurer deems a medical procedure experimental and decides not to pay for it, it completely upsets our expectations as a society. Those "noncoverage" events are so out of synch with expectations that those incidents of nonpayment for specific procedures actually become news. TV news programs report stories about incidents of noncoverage for experimental care with the same tone of outrage that they usually reserve for stories about bank fraud, trust fund embezzlement, and animal abuse.

The American way at this point in our history is to be insulated by insurance from just about all the incident-based costs of care, and Americans expect their insurance coverage to be complete. The challenge is that Americans also expect their coverage to be cheap.

The only way that most fully insured Americans today experience even an indirect cost impact of care choices is through insurance premiums. Most Americans do pay at least a portion of their insurance premium. Because managed care was able to hold health care costs flat for most of the 1990s, the out-of-pocket premium cost for most Americans has also now been flat for a very long time. That decade of flat premiums has created yet another public expectation: that there will be no increase in future health care premiums.

This particular expectation is now being turned on its ear. As health care costs rise, insurance premiums follow suit. Millions of individual Americans are already finding their personal share of premiums increasing.

That their premiums are escalating will be shocking and puzzling for most Americans. Why puzzled? Because surveys show that most people do not understand the relationship between the cost of care and the cost of premium. In fact, when asked in surveys to identify the factors that go into health care premium increases, most people rate "increasing care costs" very low on the list. Most people believe that insurance administrative expenses are the primary factor causing premium increases. They do not relate costs of care to costs of premiums. We were stunned to learn that fact, but once we learned it, a lot of very confusing aspects of most peoples' responses to premium increases became much clearer.

It's going to be difficult to hold a meaningful national policy debate about the impact of health care costs on premiums and people's take-home pay if most people literally do not link those premium increases to increases in the cost of care.

The linkage is actually pretty direct. When any insured medical procedure is performed, someone has to come up with the money to pay for it. The insurance companies or health plans usually get the credit for writing those big heart transplant checks. And the ongoing dialysis and kidney transplant checks. And the $2 million check for the McCaughey septuplets. What is overlooked is that those checks come from the premiums paid by all of the insurance companies customers. The insurers don't originate the money. They just pass the bills on.

We've all heard people say, "His insurance company paid for the whole operation. It didn't cost a penny." In fact, it did cost someone a penny. Ultimately, that someone is whoever actually pays the premium.

Insurers Are a Conduit for Cash, Not a Source

At this point, a dangerous debate is very possible. People who should be well informed truly don't understand the direct and immediate linkage between care decisions, health care costs, and insurance premiums. A national newspaper story recently asserted that the primary cause of cost increases in American health care today is the new round of premium increases being charged by insurance companies and health plans. That perspective, of course, missed the whole point completely. Where did all of those insurance premium increases come from? Free care?

So how should we more accurately describe the process of payment for health care? People need to realize that everyone who pays premiums—employers and employees—are the source of the money that pays for all care. Consumers, not insurers, actually pay for care.

The very best insurers, which are well-organized health plans, negotiate lower provider fees and improve patient care, but the premiums they charge are, in the end, simply the cost of care, divided among all premium payers.

Care Costs Create Premium Costs

The second basic fact that needs to be understood is that premiums are merely the arithmetic sum of the cost of care. When insurers write checks to fund today's wonderful array of medical miracles, they simply add up all of the costs of those miracles and then pass that cost on (proportionately) to each of their customers in the form of premiums.

It's simple arithmetic: care costs create premium costs. As care costs increase, those new costs are immediately and automatically added very directly, penny for penny, into the premium paid by each insured person.

Million Dollar Miracle

As care costs increase, it's sometimes possible to figure out how much each of us pays for individual miracles. As one example, consider that a health plan has a patient with a condition whose ongoing pharmaceutical bill exceeds a million dollars a year. Without a daily array of wonderful new drugs and chemicals, she would be dead. With them, she has the potential to live for many years. It's a miracle.

Miracles cost money for everyone, so her million-dollar-a-year drug bill is charged to all of the members. If that plan has fewer than a million members, each member would pay slightly more than a dollar a year to pay for that single patient. Every other customer and member of the plan literally pays a tiny bit of that patient's drug bill every month. All of the members, in aggregate, are keeping her alive. All should be proud and pleased to be able to do that. We all share in that miracle. We all pay for it.

Every Insured Person Pays for Every Heart Transplant

As individuals see their premiums rise and the political debate heats up, they need to remember the truth that every insured person pays for each heart transplant. The premium collected from each individual has a designated piece in it to pay for each of those transplants.

Every insured person also pays for each premature baby. And for each brain tremor implant.

Every insured person also pays for each covered prescription for Prozac, Viagra, or Prilosec.

Every single insured person pays for every mandated benefit. When a state legislature passes a law requiring that some new and untested medical procedure be covered by insurers, the cost of paying claims for that new procedure has to be passed on, proportionately and directly, to each person who pays a premium.

"Pooling" Doesn't Create New Money

Amazingly, even some very sophisticated and experienced public policy leaders too often don't understand this very basic fact. There is a nonlogical and somewhat wishful belief on the part of some lawmakers that the premiums collected by insurers are somehow magical—that the money that insurers need to pay for new mandated services doesn't have to be passed on directly as premium increases to every premium payer.

Those particular legislators never explain the mathematical magic that would allow this belief to be true. But quite a few do seem to believe it. One legislator explained to one of us that insurers would not have to increase their rates to cover a new mandated benefit because insurers actually pool their expenses. And, he said, when you pool expenses, then you can cover more things without having to raise rates.

Strange math, stranger logic. "Pooling" somehow makes money grow? That's not logical thinking; it's magical thinking. Popular magical thinking.

The American public and our leaders all need to know that pooling does not create new money. It can't. Pooling just lets the cost for each member be spread out across all members. If you increase the cost for any member, then that increased cost has to be spread across all members. So everyone, not "no one," pays for each miracle of modern medicine. Care costs are spread out, not erased, by pooling.

So, contrary to popular thinking, pooling is not an actuarial cash expansion device that can somehow make new money spring into existence. Life would be easier for a lot of people in the insurance industry if pooling did magically expand money.

When drug companies create chemical miracles and sell them to us all, who pays? All of us. Every single individual insurance customer is that payer. Each insured person pays for each newly covered drug and for every prescription drug price increase. These drug price increases are a major reason that premiums are now going up 20 percent per year. We each pay for every increase, whether or not we personally use the drug.

That's how pooling really works. It doesn't make costs disappear; it just spreads them around. We each pay a little piece of every expense. As new care costs occur, those costs are added to each member's premium every month.

Health Care Costs Are Not Distributed Evenly

Another extremely important key point to remember in looking at health care premiums is that the actual use of both health care and insurance benefits is never distributed evenly over the entire population. The fact that everyone in a given group usually pays the same premium can give people the false impression that everyone in the group uses about the same amount of care. That's not even close to true. In any given year, about 20 percent of the population incurs no health care costs at all.[1] About 70 percent of the population incurs only 10 percent of the total cost. At the other end of the continuum, 1 percent of the population incurs 30 percent of the health care costs. Five percent use over 50 percent of the total care.

Any proposed solution to the health care cost issue that does not address that cost distribution reality directly is doomed to fail. This is critically important information to understand. Everyone concerned about health care costs needs to understand this key point.

Figure 3.1 shows that distribution of actual expenses. As you look at the issue of health care costs, it's important to understand

Figure 3.1. Health Care Cost Continuum

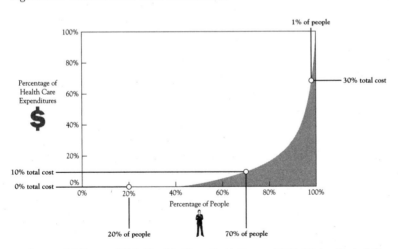

Source: Milliman USA Health Cost Guidelines—2001 Claim Probability Distributions.

that the vast majority of expenses are generated by a relatively small number of people—people with serious chronic diseases (like arthritis or diabetes) or even more serious acute illnesses (like cancer or stroke).

Health insurance premiums are usually calculated as the "weighted average" cost of care for a given group of people. That "average" number is often misunderstood by experts and the public alike to be the "usual" expense level for each citizen.

As you can see from Figure 3.2, the "premium" is simply the average cost of care, not the usual cost of care. Some people spend a lot more money on care than the premium generates. Most people spend a lot less. Each insurance pool generates a cash surplus from the people on the left side of the figure—the majority of health care consumers—but generates a huge deficit from the fewer less healthy people on the right side of the figure. If you learn no other concept from this book, that piece of information will be worth the read. It explains the economics of insurance in real terms. For insurance to work, that balance of surplus and loss has to exist. If only sick people buy coverage, there won't be any surpluses to offset the deficits.

Figure 3.2. Premium Relative to Health Care Cost Continuum

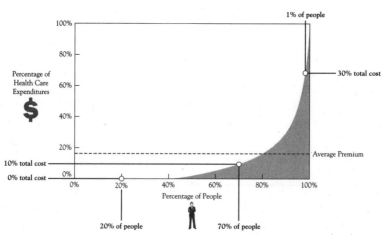

Source: Milliman USA Health Cost Guidelines—2001 Claim Probability Distributions.

Any health care reform approach, governmental or private, that somehow pulls the healthy left-side population out of the risk pool (and payment stream) is doomed to fail because each insurer would then have to calculate a new average cost amount using just the less healthy population. That sick-people-specific new premium could be two or three times higher than today's melded premium, unaffordable for almost all buyers. That approach is destined to fail as a market solution.

Focusing on Right-Hand Side of Figure 3.2 Is Critical

Any health care reform that doesn't focus on improving the care available to the people on the right-hand side of the risk continuum is also doomed to fail because that's where the real opportunities and the real expenses are. A solid, well-thought-out and well-designed program that cuts the rate of complications for diabetes, for example, has a direct impact on those right-side costs, and can help bring the total cost of care down. That, of course, would bring premiums down.

Too often, people attempting to reform health care financing miss the point entirely about where the real cost opportunities are. Too many proposals deal with the low-cost people on the left-hand side of the figure. Benefit design changes that make the 70 percent of the people who use only 10 percent of the care better users of health care services are (for obvious reasons) not the silver bullet that some people hope for. Making those 70 percent of the people 10 percent more efficient in using the care system would cut total costs by only 1 percent, not enough to make a dent in a 20 percent annual cost trend. The real focus needs to be on the high-cost people: preventing their diseases, avoiding their complications, and providing optimal care so they get well faster and receive efficient levels of services.

If employers choose to deal with overall costs by simply reducing benefits, the impact will be felt most by the people on the right-hand side of this care expense continuum—people who are facing a significant health issue and now could face a personal cost crisis as well. If the benefit reductions involve using large deductibles, those reductions will have no impact on the 20 percent of the people who now use 0 percent of the care. On the other end of the continuum, a large deductible will also have a painful but relatively brief impact on the people who are really ill and consume most of the health care expenses. A $1,000 deductible pays for only about eight hours of hospital care, for example, so the entire deductible becomes irrelevant partway through a one-day hospital stay. That front-end deductible certainly won't have a relevant decision-guiding impact on anyone who is severely ill, because it simply affects the initial cost of care, not the total cost of care.

Relying purely on a benefit-cost shift to reduce the overall costs of care will make 70 plus percent of the people unhappy with a less-than-optimal impact on the overall costs of care. The 70 percent will be particularly unhappy if the benefit costs are combined with an increase in the amount of money taken from their paycheck for health insurance premiums. At that point, the question of who pays for all of that care will become obvious to millions of Americans. When that happens, a whole new dialogue about health care costs will begin. That conversation is inevitable.

A combination of new technology, new procedures, new drugs, an aging population, health care worker wage increases, and improved negotiating leverage by consolidated health care providers is driving up care costs. When that dialogue gets under way, one of the major results will be that people will begin to think about what care we should be paying for. At that point, the whole conversation about experimental care will change.

What Impact Do Insurance Administrative Costs and Profits Have?

Surveys show that most Americans believe that insurance administrative expenses are now a primary driver for premium costs. People guess, in fact, that HMO and insurance administrative costs are

about 30 to 40 percent of premiums and that insurer profits add another 10 to 20 percent to the total cost. It is true that both insurance
companies and health plans do add an expense piece to the cost of
coverage. But the real numbers in each of those expense categories
are far different (and generally far lower) than the perceptions.
Health plan administrative costs, including profits and marketing,
average from 5 to 30 percent of total premium, depending on the
plan.[2] (A very small number of totally integrated plans, including
the ones we work for, have managed to achieve far lower numbers.)
Those percentages have been consistent for over a decade.

Ask your carrier for its specific numbers. That's a relevant and
important piece of information to know.

If the belief that plans now spend 30 to 40 percent of premiums
collected for administrative costs were true, then that would point
out a huge potential for cost savings and easy reform. Unfortunately,
or fortunately, those numbers aren't true. The real administrative
expense numbers tend to be much lower than the myth, and the administrative number generally stays at a fairly fixed level month to
month and year to year. So in spite of the widely held public misperception, administrative cost increases and plan profits are not
the major drivers of today's huge premium increases. Care costs are.
Very directly.

This doesn't mean that you should ignore either plan or insurer
administrative costs or profit levels. Consumers, buyers, policymakers, regulators, and legislators should also be very aware of what
those numbers are. The point being made here is that those expenses are not the reason that costs are going up today. Administrative costs have been relatively flat for years. It is care costs that
are exploding.

4

. . . .

If It Works or Might Work, You Owe It to Me

How Americans' Entitlement to Care Drives Up Costs

One major difference in the use of drugs and technology in the United States as compared to other countries is that most American citizens—those with private health insurance—have a personal legal right to certain drugs and procedures. America has in effect, an "entitlement" system when it comes to determining access to prescriptions and medical procedures for insured persons. We also have a strong entitlement expectation about our access to all levels of care.

By contrast, in Western countries with comprehensive government-run national health insurance programs, where only the minister of health can approve new technology or new drugs, individual citizens generally have no personal, legal, or ethical entitlement to any particular drugs, technologies, or new treatments. The government in those countries decides what is on or off the list of available medical services. The government also decides how often or extensively any care will be available. These care availability decisions are generally made based on the relative usefulness of the service and the availability of government money. The government decides how many magnetic resonance imaging (MRI) units will be available or which drugs will be used by local doctors. Individual people in those countries have no legal or ethical entitlement to use or be covered for any drugs or technologies not on the government list. People also have no right to any health care service that isn't in the current budget for that country. These budgets are, in most single-payer countries, tightly managed and rigorously enforced. In quite a few countries, a private, supplemental, nongovernment health insurance and care delivery marketplace and infrastructure has also been created, with private insurance companies selling additional levels of nongovernment coverage. Access to the separate private plans is usually limited to those citizens who personally have enough money to pay for more quickly accessible nongovernment care. These systems tend to be quite limited in scope, but have very loyal customers because the government-run insurance and care systems often leave so much to be desired for patients with serious health care problems.

The reality is that government budgets dictate the availability of care in each country with a government-run, single-payer system. As a result, in most countries with government-run health systems, a great many specialized services are in very short supply even when they represent a category of care that has been approved for inclusion in the government programs because the government doesn't have the money for more. As an example, the Canadian government decides how many MRI units will be available. There are more MRIs in Minnesota than in all of Canada. MRI wait times in Minnesota are measured in hours; wait times in Canada are measured in months, and those waiting times are getting longer, not shorter. A study published by the *Canadian Medical Association Journal* found that median waiting times in Quebec for breast cancer surgery, for example, jumped 37 percent, from twenty-nine days in 1992 to forty-two days in 1998.[1] The findings indicated that half of the women waited more than forty-two days.

Waiting times for specialty procedures in Great Britain can also be considerable. The average British patient had to wait more than twenty-nine weeks to get inpatient hospital treatment in 2000. The longest average wait was for orthopedic surgeries: nearly thirty-seven weeks.[2] In the United States, a one-week wait time for urgent orthopedic surgery is considered poor service.

Similarly, heart surgery that is available on a same-day basis in the United States can take six months to schedule in London. One recent study reports that five hundred patients die each year in London while they sit on the waiting list for routine heart operations.[3]

Roughly 50,000 British patients have waited over a year for a simple hospital admission after their doctor decided they ought to be admitted.[4] This "rationing" keeps British costs at about half of U.S. costs (7.3 percent[5] of gross domestic product as opposed to 14 percent).[6] The British health care delivery system, however, isn't anywhere near as responsive to patient needs, especially when patients are truly sick. In fact, in response to growing waiting lists, Britain's National Health Service (NHS) is increasingly turning to private hospitals in Britain. In 1998–1999, the NHS paid for about 350,000 operations in private hospitals; this number is expected to grow by about 100,000 a year.[7] Patients able to pay privately also seek care in other countries. The German embassy in London distributes brochures advertising package deals for health care that include airfare.[8] (The German system is set up very much like the managed competition model that the Clinton administration tried so hard to sell to the United States in the early 1990s.)

In nearby Scotland, nearly 200,000 Scots waited eighteen weeks or more for their first outpatient appointment in 2000.[9] In Ireland, the wait time for discretionary, nonemergency bypass surgery is over a year.

In parts of Spain, a six-month wait to have a cancer specialist review a questionable mammogram is the norm. In the United States, that would be malpractice.

Canadians often come to the United States for care not available in their country. For example, the Ontario government has a contract with private U.S. health care providers for cancer treatments for Canadians.[10] From April 1999 to April 2000, about 700 Ontario cancer patients were treated in three U.S. cities.[11]

A survey of teaching hospitals in British Columbia, Washington State, and Oregon showed that at least eighteen surgical and diagnostic procedures readily available in the United States are unavailable in Canada.[12] It's not surprising, therefore, that not only are patients leaving Canada, doctors are also leaving. There are eighteen Canadian doctors leaving permanently for the United States for every one doctor who permanently migrates from the United States to Canada.[13]

In every country with a government-run national health service, the government sets health budgets, and the health care delivery system then figures out how much care can be provided under that budget. The budgets rule supreme. They dictate care. People are not entitled to any nonbudgeted care.

By contrast, in the United States, any new technology that is shown to work and meets the standards of "medical necessity" as outlined later in the book falls immediately under a general entitlement umbrella for most insured persons. We have a huge capacity for highly technical care in this country and with minimal wait times, because people here are "entitled" to receive the care and because U.S. citizens almost always have someone else (the private insurers) pay for that care. No minister of health in Washington, D.C., decides how many MRIs or gamma knife units will exist or be used in Minneapolis, Milwaukee, Miami, or Manhattan.

In Canada, each MRI has to be approved in a legislative budgeting process. An MRI in Canada is an "expense." An MRI in the United States is a profit center. Guess which approach results in more MRIs?

MRIs are everywhere in the United States because their use is paid for by private market insurance, not by government budgets. Gamma knives don't even exist yet in the Canadian care system.

That the United States has chosen a very expensive approach to care is not necessarily bad. Why shouldn't we as a wealthy society spend money on health care technology that works? MRIs are expensive, but they are wonderful diagnostic devices. Why guess at a problem when you can simply view it?

MRIs and the other new viewing technologies represent a major change in the way conditions are diagnosed. Over the past fifty years, traditionally trained neurologists had developed an amazing set of pre-MRI skills to detect the existence of brain tumors. These "old school" doctors can do amazing diagnosis by watching the way patients' eyes follow a moving flame or by asking questions to determine certain levels of brain functioning. Those indirect diagnostic methodologies were all very ingeniously invented because it was usually far too dangerous to the patient to take a saw and knife to the skull to open up the head to look at the actual brain in search of possible clots, clogs, or tumors.

Today, an American neurologist can put the patient in a scanner and quickly and accurately use a totally noninvasive way to see exactly where in the brain an inappropriate lump, bump, or clump might be forming.

Is it better to view or to guess? It costs a couple of hundred dollars to very skillfully guess. It can cost a couple of thousand dollars to view. If you are the patient, which level of diagnosis do you want? Guess or view? That's not a hard question, but it is an expensive one. We Americans keep our MRIs very busy, and every individual's premium charge contains a piece of the cost of every scan.

One of the authors of this book had a telling conversation recently with a couple of neurology professors from a well-known medical school. They were bemoaning their inability to teach the old "follow-the-moving-finger" techniques to the new neurological residents. One teacher said the students looked at him as if he were a witch doctor.

"Why should I do all of that when I can just pop the patient into a machine and get it exactly right the first time?" he was asked. The professor didn't have an easy answer. He said he felt like a hand weaver being replaced by the steam mills of the industrial revolution.

In Canada, the moving finger is still the diagnostic technique of choice because it is much better for the provincial budget. Fingers are free. Scanners cost millions. It's an easy choice.

Is 1 Percent Worth $200,000?

A similar situation exists in cancer analysis. A skilled pathologist can put a tumor cell under a microscope and, for a $47 fee, tell us with 99 percent certainty whether the cell is malignant. That's amazing science and excellent care. It is, in fact, the best care in the world, up until now. Being 99 percent accurate still leaves a 1 percent chance that the diagnosis is wrong. We are very close, at this point, to being able to do better.

Now, with a new set of extremely sophisticated genetic code scanning equipment, that same pathologist can subject that same tumor to a detailed genetic analysis, breaking the tumor cell down to its genetic code. With this new approach, the pathologist may soon be able to tell with a higher level of certainty whether the cell is malignant. The new genetic screen costs $2,300.[14] The microscope test cost $47.

Which process should we use? If we can be 98 to 99 percent accurate with one test, is it worth another $2,000 per patient to figure out most of the final 1 percent? Should we do 99 unneeded high-tech genetic screens, at a total cost of roughly $200,000, to identify that one additional cancer case, one additional malignancy?

If you are the one in a hundred patients whose cancer might have otherwise gone undetected, do you think the $200,000 in diagnostic testing will be worth spending?

Today, the best standard of care in the world says that 99 percent accuracy is good enough. But the pressure will very quickly be on to do the additional screens and spend the additional money. If that happens, the cost of each test will be an added cost for each premium payment by each member.

To complicate that example a bit more, a prominent oncologist who has looked at that new genetic screening process believes it will soon give him a whole new range of tumor-specific data that will let him do a much better job of identifying the exact type of cancer involved. If that's true, he believes he will be able to treat each individual cancer patient with a higher degree of success. Does this make the test worth $2,000 per patient?

These kinds of developments in care are wonderful miracles, and in this country they come as part of the overall package of entitlement for patients. The impact of patient entitlement to all proven care is a constant expansion of the scope of care. When medical technology development companies know that they can get their new devices paid for if they are proved to work, then those companies have both a guaranteed market and a guaranteed payer, so of course they are always developing more technology.

As one might expect, the dual impact of these economic factors is a constant improvement in care and a constant expansion in the cost of that care.

No One Collects a Penny for "Unproven" Care Coverage

Challenging as it is, paying for proven care is not the most difficult issue we face today. The real difficulty is how to deal with "unproven" care. It's somewhat easy to argue that insurers should pay for very expensive technology as long as the care is known to work. But what about extremely expensive technology that is still experimental, and therefore unproven? What if no one knows whether a particular treatment has any real likelihood of working? Should we pay huge sums of money from our insurance premium for unproven care?

Surveys show that Americans clearly feel entitled to be treated with unproven technologies as well as proven. Most Americans want everything to be covered, whether or not there is any valid evidence that the care works. In one survey done a few years ago, people were asked whether a health plan should spend a million dollars to provide experimental care to attempt to save the life of a newborn baby if there was only a 1 percent chance that the care would work. Ninety percent of the people surveyed said, "Spend the money." A 1 percent chance was worth a million dollars to the people surveyed. It was, at least, worth a million dollars of "other people's money." No one was asked how much in extra premium he or she would be willing to pay or if that 1 percent possibility of success would have been worth writing a personal check for a million dollars. In any case, Americans clearly want insurance to cover expensive, experimental care, even if the likelihood of success is relatively small.

Technology companies and pharmaceutical manufacturers naturally agree with the public. They run ads encouraging patients to demand coverage for clinical trials from their insurers and health plans. The ads don't mention that the technology companies and pharmaceutical manufacturers will receive billions of dollars in premium money if they succeed in getting those procedures covered.

That raises an interesting issue: How should we pay for experimental, unproven care? The long-standing tradition of American health coverage is to pay for all proven care but not for experimental care. The official policy-based thinking on that topic has been that experiments of that sort should be done in controlled settings, using careful levels of scientific rigor, and that academic, government, or technology company money should be used to pay for those experiments instead of private insurance money.

Insurance was not designed, written, or priced to cover experiments.

That can create real problems when patients with insurance coverage want to use their coverage to pay for experimental treatments. Insurers respond by saying they cover only proven care, not all possible care. In fact, no insurer, to the best of our knowledge, now sells coverage for unproven treatments. All insurance policies that we know of very specifically exclude "experimental and unproven care" from coverage.

Because these benefits are excluded, no insurer today collects a penny of premium to pay for experimental care. If insurers covered experimental care, that would necessitate premium increases. Those additional premiums have not been billed or collected, so insurers generally believe they have no obligation to provide coverage that no one paid for. That fact, however, doesn't change the sense that most Americans have that they are entitled to that experimental care. Most believe that their premium did, in fact, include a charge for experimental services. There is a remarkable lack of societal clarity on that issue.

This difference of perspective has created one of the most heated, visible, and controversial issues in American health care: Should entitlement extend to experiments? Should all carriers increase their coverage (and premiums) to cover experimental care?

On this issue, the news media clearly and consistently disagree with the insurers' position and believe strongly that untested and unproven care should be covered. Newspapers and TV news shows regularly run highly emotional and deeply indignant stories when any level of care or coverage is denied. They never say in those stories, "XYZ health plan has never collected a penny of premium to pay for experimental care, but we think they should cover it anyway." The media often ignore both insurance contract language and even a complete lack of medical evidence for a specific item of care. Instead they say, "XYZ health plan is letting Ann Smith die because the plan refuses to pay for the care she needs." Or "XYZ health plan is keeping this child from developing fully because they refuse to pay for water immersion therapy for this child."

In quite a few cases, even a complete and total lack of scientific support for the requested care is not considered to be relevant when those stories are told to the public. In some cases, the only vocal public advocates for the experimental care approach are the very same people who have invented the care, own the care site, and stand to make a lot of money providing it, whether or not it works. Some members of the media tend to use quotations from those highly biased sources as if their opinions had only scientific validity, not personal financial or academic self-interest.

Every reader of this book has seen those news stories. The public has no way of knowing what is true, so the public tends to side with the dramatic perspective of condemning the carrier for not providing the unproven care.

Relaxing Standards and Rising Costs

Why is this topic covered in a book on rising health care costs? Because media and consumer pressure to cover experimental care is creating another cost pressure of its own. Because of the pressure, the level of rigor used to define experimental care has been significantly loosened in recent years. Because of this relaxed rigor, unproven, untested experimental care does get covered in some cases. These costs are being added to everyone's premium. They're one of today's relevant cost drivers.

That's just the immediate impact. The future impact on costs could be much larger. Expanding coverage to cover all experimental care would open the door to expense increases that will result directly in much greater premium increases for each of us.

That's an issue that needs to be discussed. The perspectives are pretty clear. That coverage expansion is what consumers currently want—at least until the price impact on premiums is felt. Consumers want the benefits. Providers want the cash flow and the profits. Insurers want to cover what works, not unproven experiments. The American expectation of fully entitled coverage for every possible approach to care is amazingly strong, so the leaning right now is in the direction of increasing expenses, premiums, and coverage.

So how can we resolve that situation? Who should pay for experimental care?

The traditional third-party payer expectation in this country, and the long-standing expectation of government programs like Medicare and Medicaid, is that unproven experimental care should be funded only by academic grants and research moneys, until that wonderful moment in the research process when the value of the care is actually proven. Once proven, insurers should pay. Everyone agrees that care that actually works should be, and is, covered. Once proven, each new procedure is now immediately paid for by just about all forms of standard insurance.

The media and public tend to take a different perspective, urging the expansion of coverage to include all experimental care, regardless of the current level of scientific evidence about the value of the experiments.

How About Paying Only for Experiments That Work?

Some novel payment approaches have been tried for experimental care. A few plans have said to medical researchers, "Try it. If it works, we'll pick up the bill. If it fails, then it's your cost, not ours."

That seems to be a reasonable compromise. On that basis, covering experimental care would be a snap. Most insurers would do it in a microsecond. But most medical researchers know that most research fails. So having their personal incomes tied to the actual success of their unproven care isn't at all attractive to most research professionals.

There is some irony in the fact that the same researchers who enthusiastically extend hope to individual patients are, almost without exception, far too practical about the actual value of their experimental care to risk their own income on its success.

The University of Minnesota Medical School is an inspiring exception to that rule. It has been willing to tie success to dollars in a number of experimental cases. That approach has been a win for researchers, insurers, and patients.

In any case, most insurers have loosened their definitions of experimental care in recent years in part because of public attitudes and in part because courts in the United States increasingly rule in favor of consumers who want experimental care. Judges and juries like possible miracles as much as anyone else.

And, to be fair, the result of that relaxation of rigor has been additional miracles in at least a few cases. The miracles are often expensive, but they are miracles nonetheless. Some experiments do work. That's good, particularly if you are the patient.

What Happens When Lawyers and Legislatures Practice Medicine?

In other cases, the results of using unproven medical procedures because of public or legal pressure have been disastrous. The laws enacted in state after state a couple of years ago mandating insurance coverage for autologous bone marrow transplants for breast cancer patients are a case in point.

These laws were all well meaning. The legislators who wrote the laws, however, ignored the rather obvious scientific fact that no researcher had proven anywhere in any setting that those transplants actually worked. One slightly biased study using healthier-than-average patients indicated that the treatment might possibly work. Over time, even the patients in that study died. But science wasn't the issue. Hope trumped science. Politics trumped policy. Good-hearted lawmakers everywhere, in the hopes that the transplants might work, legally mandated them.

Elected officials were not alone in their enthusiasm for these particular experiments. In several states where legislatures did not mandate the transplants, the courts did. Dozens of court cases forced plans everywhere to pay for these unproven treatments. Legislatures, lawyers, and judges freely played doctor.

The results? Pain. Suffering. Isolation. Failure. Death.

Large-scale scientific tests have since proven fairly conclusively that the legally mandated bone marrow transplant procedure may have been very profitable for many of the caregivers involved, but it did not work to help breast cancer patients. (A few caregiving institutions, to their great shame, continued doing the highly profitable procedure in large volumes for quite a while after it was proven to be useless.)

Until the definitive effectiveness studies were completed on the use of bone marrow transplants for breast cancer, many thousands of women received the unproven treatment and died unnecessarily miserable and even gruesome deaths. Bone marrow transplants are an excruciating, risk-filled procedure. The whole point of the procedure is to extract the patient's bone marrow and put it in safekeeping so the rest of the body can be subjected to otherwise high levels of poisons and radiation with the intent of killing the cancers. To the patient, the whole process is painful and very dangerous. The treatment itself clearly shortened some lives.

While being treated, the patients had to be temporarily isolated from the people they loved to protect them from infection. Being kept apart from the people they loved in the little time they had to live was a terrible extra emotional burden for these women. It's particularly sad when that isolation added no value to their care.

The women who were subjected to this aggressive treatment then died at similar rates as other women who were given normal cancer treatments, but with higher levels of pain and suffering and with less contact with their loved ones. Some women in fact died much earlier because the treatment itself was high risk.

Health Plans Wanted That Procedure to Work

It would have been wonderful if the treatment had worked. Another miracle would have become available. We very much need better treatments for Stage Four breast cancers. No one disputes that fact.

In fact, before any laws were passed about the procedure, Health-Partners had been evaluating careful clinical trials to see if this particular treatment for breast cancer worked. Those scientific trials were impaired when the legal mandates began, because it was difficult to recruit women. The control groups and the studies lost their scientific validity.

In any of these countries where the government rigorously applies the standard that says a treatment must be proven to work before it can be used widely, that tragic episode of painful and useless care would never have happened.

The phen-fen debacle was similar. A large number of patients heard through various sources that a combination of phentermine and fenfluramine (both drugs developed for other medical purposes) could help people lose weight. There was some science to back that claim, but, more important, no clinical trials had revealed significant side effects or completely evaluated safety and there was a high level of patient demand. The medical grapevine said phen-fen worked. The Internet said phen-fen worked. Many doctors listened to their patients' requests, ignored the lack of research, and wrote the prescriptions.

Most health plans and insurers invoked their "experimental therapy" exclusions and refused to cover that use of those particular drugs. Many patients protested that plan decision both privately and publicly, calling the insurers cheap and heartless, until subsequent Mayo Clinic research showed that the drugs were severely damaging some patients.

We Need Research to Find Tomorrow's Miracles

Sometimes medical miracles don't happen even when everyone has the best intentions. That's why careful research is necessary; we need experiments to figure out how to achieve the next generation of miraculous care. Every year, solid medical research produces additional wins and adds to the proven medical tool kit. It's an increasingly big kit. Transplants, eye surgeries, implants, and beta ray surgery all now add great value to people's lives. None of us is willing to roll back the clock and return to the level of technology, skill, drugs, and care available in 1990—not even to get 1990 care prices.

We could easily cut today's health care costs by 20 percent or more by eliminating all drugs and technologies invented since 1990. But no one familiar with the new tool kit for care would make that choice. We get the miracles. We want the miracles. We refuse to ration miracles. Our system makes people entitled to the miracles. So we all have to pay the price.

We all need to recognize that the current arrays of modern medical miracles, dramatic as they are, are just the tip of the iceberg. We are nearing a time where genetic science will allow us to detect disease earlier and treat it much more effectively. We will be able to modify genes in living people. We will be able to develop and target drugs based on people's personal gene configuration. People will benefit immediately, and significantly.

Costs will, of course, skyrocket.

What will fund this expanding universe of new treatments? Premiums! Premiums paid by us all.

Anyone who looks at medical science can predict, without question, that we as a society will see huge additional cost pressures resulting from medical technology and pharmaceutical science. When those miracles happen and they work, we all will pay.

Employers now pay the bulk of health insurance premiums for most Americans. As costs surge, premiums follow. Many employers are now telling us that they can't afford to pay the total of cost increases for their employees. Those employers are also beginning to challenge the whole concept of full entitlement to all care for their employees. Those employers will have hard decisions to make. They will either drop coverage altogether, forcing their employees to become uninsured, or the employers will shift many of the increased costs to their employees.

As individual employees see benefit drops and decreases in their take-home pay, the whole issue of entitlement to benefits will become the topic of discussion at many levels. If they must share in the cost, some people will make decisions about benefit use very differently. Therapies that consumers demand when they are fully covered by insurers, and therefore "free," may suddenly be in lower demand when the patient has to pay a relevant and proportionate portion of the cost.

Some employers are also choosing to self-insure so they can avoid paying for some state-mandated benefits. Federal law allows self-insured employers to avoid compliance with some state benefit laws. If either courts or legislators increase insurer liability for experimental care, the number of employers switching to self-insurance will grow even more quickly.

These issues are all discussed in more detail in the final chapters of this book. For now, suffice it to say that the golden age of full entitlement is still in full bloom, and the result has been to help create the health care cost trends we all face.

That golden age may soon be only a golden memory for many underinsured *and* uninsured people.

5

Care Monopolies

Hospital fees charged to health plans and insurance companies have increased by 20 to 50 percent in many markets over the past couple of years. Those cost increases flow directly to member premium increases. How did hospitals get into position to charge those levels of increase? A quick review of health plan provider contracting history is useful to understand the current problem.

A very small number of health plans, including Kaiser Permanente, HealthPartners, and Group Health of Puget Sound, deliver a substantial portion of their care through exclusive networks of physicians closely allied with, if not employed by, the plan. In those settings, fees were not and are not the mechanism for physician payment. In most health plan situations, however, fees are the primary way both doctors and hospitals are paid, and through the 1990s, health plans negotiated hard to reduce those fees.

In fact, one of the major reasons for the remarkable health care cost stability of the 1990s was the ability and willingness of those contracting health plans to use volume purchasing leverage to reduce the fees charged by providers. Those plans, in other words, negotiated deep discounts—30 to 50 percent discounts in many cases. These discounts cut health plan costs to the point that most plans could significantly underprice the old pre-HMO traditional insurance products. Traditional health insurance organizations usually didn't have comparable fee discounts, so they had to pay claims at full retail price levels. That made their premiums much less competitive than HMO premiums. Consumers benefited directly from the negotiated fee discounts because those discounts allowed health plans to cut premium levels.

Providers of care were not happy about those fee cuts. Those discounts significantly reduced the amount of money going to physicians, drug companies, and hospitals for each unit of care.

Doctors, very understandably, hated those lower prices. Hospitals resented them. Drug companies were deeply alarmed. All grew to intensely dislike the health plans that were paying the discounted prices.

American consumers, however, benefited tremendously from these major discounts, which sometimes exceeded 50 percent of pre-HMO provider fees. Plans in that era of deep discounts could offer richer benefits for significantly less money. It was a golden age for patients and health plans and a shocking, financially painful dark age for a great many care providers.

Much of providers' passionate dislike of health plans is linked directly (and logically) to the fact that many plans used their negotiating power without mercy against both physicians and hospitals. Those negotiations deeply cut hospital revenue along with physician cash flow. Caregiver personal incomes suffered.

It makes sense, of course, to be unhappy with any organization or economic strategy that benefits financially by cutting your personal income. It would be strange, in fact, if providers didn't dislike the plans that had cut their income.

To put the situation into a very real perspective, consider this. If you were a doctor who owned an MRI machine and if your pre-HMO retail price for a single MRI scan used to be $1,200, how would you feel about an HMO negotiator who came into your office and told you, "We've got several competing MRI bids here. Your current prices are way out of line. If you charge us more than $400 a scan, our HMO network doctors will send all of our 200,000 local patients elsewhere. So do you want to be in our network or not? If not, kiss your referrals from our doctors good-bye." Who wouldn't resent those fee cuts?

The pre-HMO $1,200 fee for an individual MRI scan had been extremely profitable. By contrast, $400 per scan is at best a break-even price. So why did any doctors sign those HMO price-cut contracts? Because there was an oversupply of MRIs in many markets and the providers who owned those machines did not want to lose patient volume. Their accountants told them that the deeply discounted $400 fee still covered all of their variable costs for each patient and at least helped offset some of their fixed costs. Most MRI owners reluctantly and angrily agreed to the discounts, getting their profits from non-HMO patients. Those that didn't accept the discounts lost patients to those that did. Competitive forces worked just as they should: true competition brought prices down.

Those discounted fees meant a major savings for the health plans. Savings of that type across many types of care providers were so good they kept HMO and preferred provider organization (PPO) premium prices flat through most of the 1990s. As the HMOs grew, their negotiating leverage increased, and their discounts grew with them. First-year 10 percent discounts sometimes ended up 50 percent discounts over four to five years.

American workers benefited because they got to keep their raises each year instead of using them to subsidize rising health care fees and premiums.

What would have happened to American workers' take-home pay in the 1990s if health plans had not negotiated those discounts? That's an important question to ask in the context of today's prices.

Keep in mind that all care-related cost pressures continued to push upward during the 1990s. New drugs and new technologies relentlessly created new expenses every single year. People aged. The demand for care increased every single year. But those ongoing upward cost pressures were all offset and hidden for years by the constantly increasing, volume-leveraged HMO discounts in provider fees and by a few basic steps that plans took to eliminate obviously wasteful care.

Health plans combined deep discounts with the kinds of externally imposed care efficiencies outlined in Chapter Seven to stabilize premium levels. Couple those price saving discounts with the HMOs' new ability to eliminate significant levels of unnecessary hospital use, and it's easy to see why the overall health care premium cost trend was actually flat through most of the 1990s, even though the complexity levels and inherent cost of care increased every single year.

Rebasing Unit Prices Created a Decade of Flat Premiums

We were all lulled by that flat premium trend into a false sense of comfort on the cost issue. Those early efficiency achievements and the heavy-handed price negotiations helped to offset and cover up the increased costs of new drugs and new technologies for the better part of a decade.

A lot of otherwise well-informed people actually looked only at total premium levels year-to-year and speculated that managed care had somehow succeeded in truly bringing overall health care cost trends permanently under control. They were wrong.

In truth, the overall care pricing system simply rebased itself on the new lower provider fees and shorter hospital stays. Discounts, however, have their limits: 100 percent discounts are not economically feasible. So when those discount fees and length-of-stay levels hit rock bottom, all of the other underlying pressures from drugs, technology, aging, and so on began to be more visible. Total costs then began once again to increase visibly. In today's provider world, those provider fee discounts are beginning to shrink, so premium increases are again becoming extremely visible and painful.

But for a while, premiums were flat, and everyone in America got used to flat premiums. Consumers and employers both thanked HMOs in the early 1990s for increasing benefits while stabilizing costs. Even journalists celebrated the HMO industry's seemingly magical ability to expand coverage while holding the line on premium. But that sense of accomplishment and goodwill lasted for only a couple of years. Then people got used to flat premiums, grew to expect them, and began to focus negatively on some of the tools health plans used to keep premiums flat.

Plans Didn't Explain the Discounts to Consumers

Any significant level of consumer gratitude for the HMO industry's remarkable cost stabilization success was relatively short-lived. The gratitude came with an inherent limitation. Consumers liked the new premium stability, but quite a few health plan members grew to strongly dislike the provider network restrictions that created the price stability. American consumers don't like being told where to receive their care. For obvious reasons, only providers that accepted the managed care discounts were included in the plan networks; providers that insisted on being paid full retail fees were not. HMO members are usually limited to receiving care from providers who are under contract to the plan.

That created a couple of problems with consumers. Americans are not fond of restrictions. A great many consumers did not like their HMO directing them to get their MRI scan from Dr. Jones instead of Dr. Smith. And then, reinforcing their unhappiness, when patients went to their new doctor for care, they often encountered an unhappy, deeply discontented (and deeply discounted) doctor. Too often, as they received care, they heard Dr. Jones curse the HMOs that were "cutting the quality of care."

That "quality reduction" language was often simply angry doctor code for "cutting my fees." Consumers couldn't detect that particular issue because they knew nothing about the actual scope or the real extent of the fee cuts. The criticisms were taken at face value. HMO credibility suffered a lot.

Interestingly, HMOs with deeply discounted contracts didn't make much of an effort to help their own cause in these situations. They never told patients about the discounts. They never explained to patients how the discounts helped keep premiums affordable.

That was a major mistake by the plans. People can't be expected to appreciate an invisible benefit. Plans seldom, if ever, tried to win consumer support by explaining that consumer premiums were flat in the 1990s largely because of those provider contracts. They didn't tell consumers about the actual cost factors or fee cuts. No one in the HMO world publicly discussed the direct relationship between those deep discounts and lower premiums, so the public never understood what was generally the most stress-provoking issue for many doctors: deep and painful provider fee cuts.

Why were HMOs silent on that key point? Primarily because individual HMOs didn't want either policymakers or other HMOs to learn how remarkably good their own discounts were. The discounts were considered to be trade secrets. Most provider contracts, in fact, had strong language requiring both parties to keep those discounts secret.

So consumers were never told, for example, "This hospital takes care of you for one thousand dollars a day. The other hospital across the street provides the same services and wants two thousand dollars a day. Paying two thousand dollars would be a waste of your money and would double your premium. That's why we use Ocean-view instead of Bayview for your hospital care."

"Care Denial" Became the Public Explanation for Plan Success

Those conversations never took place. Those letters to members were never written. So because of HMO silence on this point, consumers heard only one side of the story for a very long time: the providers' side. Consumers therefore did not and could not appreciate the plan-negotiated fee savings or support the HMOs in their extremely important role as volume-based purchasing agents because most consumers didn't even know that role existed.

So what did consumers believe plans did to keep down the costs of care? They believed plans achieved that cost control by simply "denying care." Care denial was the explanation given to consumers by many care providers—even though HMO benefits were actually far richer than the traditional insurance plans that HMOs replaced. Consumers have no clue that most of the initial cost savings of the past decade for most health plans actually came from getting a lower price for care.

Almost all caregivers, of course, knew where the real HMO savings came from. But very few doctors or hospitals wanted that information to be public either. One reason for the two-sided confidentiality contracts on fee pricing was that the typical MRI owner (or hospital or surgeon) didn't want other HMOs or care providers knowing what discounts that particular caregiver was giving to each payer.

Everyone in the provider world was afraid that every payer would demand the best deal if these deals became public knowledge. They were probably right. Health plan negotiators would have used that information to get better deals from individual providers if they had learned the providers had given "better" discounts to another plan.

Negotiating Leverage Shifted

The deeply discounted, highly leveraged purchase of health care services came with two dangerous levels of built-in, self-limiting instability for health plans. The one-sided price negotiations turned providers into enemies. It's always bad to have enemies. It's particularly bad when you need those enemies to be a key part of your product.

An even bigger long-range problem was that the deep discounts strongly encouraged providers to consolidate into larger organizations to create their own negotiations leverage. So not only did many providers continuously undermine the credibility of health plans in conversations with their patients, an increasing number of providers also finally figured out how to form the kind of local care monopolies and oligopolies that could help providers regain control of pricing. It took a number of years, but the new provider strategies to achieve price leveraging that we now see in the marketplace are exactly what economist Adam Smith would have predicted.

The Key to Controlling Price
Is to Control Supply

Doctors and hospital administrators did not like being forced to lower prices. They sat back to analyze the situation and in city after city said, "We seem to be at the mercy of the large health plans in negotiating fees. They control our patients. If we don't give them big discounts, they'll take our patients away. How can we counterattack and regain control over our fees?"

One simple answer in any supply-and-demand situation in any industry is for the seller to somehow get control over the prices by regaining control over supply. That is an ancient and generally successful economic strategy. After a decade of deep discounts, caregivers finally figured out that when there were hundreds of competing caregivers in a given market, they were all subject to price-lowering competition. Competition hurt each provider's ability to raise fees. Competition very effectively kept provider prices down in fact. If any care vendor in a highly competitive caregiver marketplace chose not to accept the plan discounts, another local physician group or hospital would happily accept the lower price and take its patients.

Competition among multiple providers in each local market worked well for the plans and their members. It did not work well for the economic interests of each independent caregiver.

If, however, providers could somehow merge into some form of local care monopoly or local, basically noncompetitive care oligopoly, then the health plans' negotiating leverage could be diminished, maybe even broken. Prices and fees could once again go up to very profitable levels for the providers.

Providers Merged to Offset Health Plan Leverage

Economic wars are won with economic weapons. Provider mergers started. All over the country, providers started acquiring other providers. Hospitals bought clinics. Clinics acquired hospitals. Hospitals merged with other hospitals. Medical groups merged with one another. Huge regional medical groups formed in some markets. All of that activity was, at its heart, a strong and effective strategic response to the growing negotiating power of local health plans.

Mergers: The Early Years

The provider merger strategy required some fine-tuning before it achieved any appreciable success. Initial efforts at merging provider businesses sometimes misfired. Quite a few backfired. Some initial mergers failed entirely.

The first provider mergers tended to not work very well, because, for the most part, they were often complex, multidisciplinary vertical mergers. They attempted to link doctors, hospitals, nursing homes, and other providers into centrally owned care systems, all with common management, common strategies, and a common bottom line. These vertical mergers were an attempt by local hospitals or clinics to copy Kaiser Permanente, the old Harvard Community Health Plan, Group Health of Minnesota, Group Health of Puget Sound, and other historically successful health plans. Those plans worked with an exclusive set of doctors, often owned their own hospitals, and managed to achieve some real efficiencies by having their doctors and hospitals function as a team.

No One Had a Clue About How to Integrate Care

When well designed and well executed, these kinds of vertically integrated care systems can have an immense positive impact on care.

This model, done well, allows all caregivers serving a given patient to function as a team. In theory, team members can focus on the patient rather than functioning as an array of separate, uncoordinated, entirely independent businesses, each seeking to maximize its own revenue under their own leadership. In a truly vertically integrated system, the doctor, hospital, and nursing home could all work together as a unit to figure out the best site and type of care for each patient without having to worry about which level or site of care received what amount of revenue.

That was the theory anyway. It really only worked well in those very few systems that had been created from the ground up to function in exactly that way. It seldom worked well in large and complex merger settings, where multiple, formerly fiercely independent caregivers suddenly found themselves forced, often against their will, onto the same corporate "team."

For starters, almost no one in any of those force-melded settings really knew how to integrate care. The theory wasn't supported by any known practice. No one teaches care integration. No one from the merged organizations knew what these very complex multilevel care teams were actually supposed to do once they were formed. Everyone knew the rhetoric, but no one knew the hard facts of life about care coordination, joint planning, and team-based care.

It all looked easy when Kaiser Permanente did it, so local hospitals and clinics thought they could do it too just by merging.

They were wrong.

The glowing rhetoric of the initial premerger press conferences held by the newly linked providers seldom matched the cold reality of the postmerger provider interactions. The strategy of merging into totally consolidated megasystems had great momentum for several years, however. Few things are more powerful than a wrong idea whose time has come.

Huge care systems formed in city after city. Then the new megasystems tried to figure out how to go forward. No one actually knew, so people inside each organization very naturally began to bicker internally about next steps. Once fully formed, the largest mega-systems tended to do amazingly bloody battle within their own walls rather than compete externally for patients. Each type, category, and level of caregiver inside those monoliths (literally hundreds were formed across the country during the 1990s) tended to be territorial, jealous, suspicious, and financially competitive with each of the other internal working parts of their own newly merged megaorganizations.

Internal battles for budget and political power became incredibly intense in many of the new vertical integration settings. Internal competition for budget was often far more intense than external competition for patients in many sites.

Adding Layers of Bureaucracy Is Not the Same as Achieving Efficiencies of Scale

To add insult to injury, many of the new vertical systems found themselves at an actual competitive disadvantage in their communities. Rather than controlling the local market, as they had hoped, they often discovered that they now had to compete for patients in an even more competitive market, going toe-to-toe with other new megasystems. Unless the new vertical entity absolutely controlled all relevant care in a total geographical area, it still had to compete for health plan patients with various other equally ambitious local caregivers. If the other local caregivers were small, they were often strategically far more nimble than the megasystems. If local competitors were large, they were needy. They all had huge payrolls and needed major flows of cash to survive. That need for cash flow created major provider system price wars. Big systems need patient volume, and that volume need often caused directly competing larger new systems to significantly underprice their services in order to achieve and maintain critical economic mass.

Health plans benefited from the providers' need for huge patient volume. Plans had the patients whom the providers needed, so plans

got the prices they wanted. Provider price wars in that era of dueling megaprovider systems helped keep plan premiums down.

To make matters even worse for the merged organizations, the
huge, crudely consolidated mega-entities typically also found themselves heavily burdened with new layers of administrative, structural, and executive overhead—often to the point that their aggregate
competitive financial position was actually impaired, rather than
improved, by what everyone in health care now knows are almost
always mythical postmerger "efficiencies of scale."

That particular term, *efficiencies of scale*, also consistently showed
up in just about all of the extremely optimistic premerger press re-
leases, but that concept rarely manifested itself as a benefit in actual financial reports provided in subsequent years by the merged
organizations.

Adding layers of management is not the same thing as achieving efficiencies of scale.

True Monopolies, Even Local Ones, Generally Triumph

There was, and is, a significant exception to the typical somewhat
counterproductive and generally dysfunctional outcome that usually results from attempts to create vertically integrated health systems. From the providers' perspective, some mergers worked very
well. Some did, in fact, give providers the exact financial leverage
and market control that they wanted. Megamergers worked extremely well indeed for providers of care in those specific situations
where actual care monopolies resulted for given geographical areas.
In many rural areas or smaller cities where true total care monopolies were achieved as the result of mergers, the new local megacare
system found itself quickly in clover. Some megaprovider organizations literally owned the total local medical care delivery infrastructure. Therefore, the providers in those systems once again
controlled both care delivery and the local pricing of care. Plans do

not like that particular outcome. It transferred economic leverage and market power from the plan to the monopoly care system in those local geographical areas. Any insurer or health plan that wanted to do business in those fully consolidated geographical areas needed to make a deal with the new care monopoly or be cut out of business in that market.

Most health plans and insurers are highly vulnerable to massive provider consolidations. Whenever providers control the delivery of care and a significant geographical area, then plans are forced to treat those providers very differently. This is most obvious in rural areas, but it's true in large cities as well.

How can provider mergers create leverage in large cities? In large communities, most employers will purchase coverage only from health plans that have a provider network that covers all of the places where their employees might live. That means big city plans can't afford to have major holes in their local networks. That need on the part of the payers to have a local provider agreement every-where in the local geography has recently allowed relatively small local care monopolies to increase fees significantly.

Monopolies Create Enough Internal Cash to Heal Internal Wounds

Another positive outcome for truly monopolistic vertically inte-grated care providers is that internal turf and budget battles within those new market-dominant megasystems often disappear. Mini-mally, those disputes are much less heated than in most other non-monopoly mergers. Why? Because monopoly megasystems can simply salve over the incessant, inevitable, and inherent internal interdepartmental battles inside their merged corporate walls by "bribing" everyone. Money heals a lot of internal organizational wounds. Market control brings revenue control. Revenue control increases cash flow. Rich new flows of cash can be used to cover up an awful lot of internal turf fighting and political dissension.

Monopoly negotiating leverage can create very rich flows of cash. Prices to consumers go up, and the morale of the caregivers goes up even more.

So mergers do work for the providers once they achieve substantial domination in a local market. Those mergers will probably be in place two decades from now.

In many of the nonmonopoly markets, however, the same care systems that enthusiastically spent the first half of the 1990s vertically integrating spent the last quarter of the decade energetically disintegrating. In many markets, that raveling and then unraveling process took up the full energy of the providers for most of the 1990s and let the local health plans maintain their market leverage and purchasing power.

Horizontal Mergers Are Easier to Do

Vertical integration wasn't the only form of merger that care providers attempted. Horizontal integration was also a popular strategy in many areas of the country. Horizontal mergers bring together all of the hospitals in an area, or all of the proctologists, or all of the allergists. Those specialty-specific mergers are easier to do, easier to manage, and easier to use as leverage to get control over specific sets of fees.

In some areas of the country, a variation of horizontal integration momentum took the form of huge medical individual practice associations (IPAs)—networks of physicians formed to provide care for various PPOs and HMOs. That particular form of horizontal consolidation has some real difficulties being successful as a way of increasing physician income. Instead of creating monopolies that let providers control local fees, many of the IPAs ventured full tilt into direct competition with each other. The IPAs usually competed with one another for local HMO business, often accepting HMO payment levels far below their costs in order to keep each local IPA's market share strong. That approach put quite a few individual providers into very poor financial condition. Again, vigorous price competition hurt that version of consolidated providers. Those fiercely competitive IPAs are now either failing or are restructuring or reorganizing in an attempt to achieve local geographical dominance.

In either case, costs are going up for both the surviving IPAs and the health plans that use them. As a result, the absolute price increase needs of the IPA physicians have recently forced HMO premiums up in a number of areas.

Toward the end of the 1990s, many caregivers finally figured out how the actual relevant marketplace worked. They realized that the two primary vulnerabilities of health plans are that (1) plans need to have adequate and broad geographical coverage to be attractive to buyers and (2) plans need to include every type of care to be attractive to patients. A health plan with an important void on its provider map tended to be less marketable. A plan that totally lacked local oncologists or dermatologists or some other essential category of care was a plan that was much less marketable. A plan totally without hospital providers in any given market was dead. Once you understand that reality, then provider strategies become self-evident if the goal is to increase provider income and revenue per patient.

Competition Doesn't Help Providers Make Money; Eliminating Competition Does

These particular slow-developing insights on the part of provider strategists were ultimately extremely useful and powerful to provider business entities in many communities. The key question still was, "How do we, as providers, put ourselves in the position to be needed by the health plans and insurers?" The new answer wasn't to be more competitive. It was to be much *less* competitive. Adam Smith could have saved the provider world a lot of time. Many providers finally realized that their ultimate financial victory in the new managed care era would come from eliminating competition, not excelling at it.

So providers in many markets in the mid- to late 1990s began to form specialty-specific horizontal mergers, designed to create monopolies around a particular type or level of care. Adjacent hospitals merged all over the country. Many major cities that used to have dozens of competing hospitals now have only one, two, or, at most, three merged and consolidated systems. Milwaukee, Boston, St. Louis, St. Paul, San Diego, San Francisco, and Salt Lake City: the pattern is very clear. Bring enough hospitals together to dominate any significant part of a local geographical market, and over a very short period of time, the price negotiation balance will shift away from the health plan and back to the local monopoly provider.

The equation is amazingly simple. For American health care consumers, it is also very expensive.

In a premerger, highly competitive hospital market, where several hospitals are each willing to give a low price to keep from losing patients, each individual hospital needs the local health plan as a source of patients, so the health plan can buy care at a lower price. In contrast, in a fully consolidated (and therefore newly noncompetitive) local hospital market, each health plan needs the merged hospital system in order to have a viable insurance product. So merged and market-dominant hospitals can dictate the local price. And they *never* dictate a lower price. It's never lower, even when the premerger rhetoric talks about "efficiencies of scale."

In other words, the "need" balance shifts when hospitals merge. As street economists say, "Whoever gots the needs pays the price."

The ultimate victim or beneficiary of those two very different negotiating worlds is the patient. When the plans were winning (because multiple hospitals were competing with each other), premium prices to consumers went down. Premium, remember, is the arithmetic sum of the cost of care. And when the newly consolidated hospital systems win and increase their charges, premium prices to consumers simply go up.

When plan discounts shrink, patient costs expand. The math is pretty simple.

Keep in mind that the hospitals are facing their own huge cost pressures. Technology costs are exploding. Staff costs are exploding. Federal and state governments are cutting reimbursement levels to the point of real financial pain. These government payment cuts have put major pressure on the hospitals to shift costs whenever possible to private market payers. The hospitals are not villains in this equation, but they definitely have moved upstream on the negotiating leverage.

Specialist Mergers Are Easy to Build and Can Be Financially Very Rewarding

A similar pattern of consolidation and price increase is also occurring in specialty care. In one recent example, when just about all of a particular specialty that provided care to a number of hospitals stopped competing and merged into one big group for an entire geographical area, the price paid for that care shot up overnight. One-hour therapy jumped by 51 percent premerger to postmerger. A hospital follow-up visit increased by 20 percent. Multiple-hour therapy more than doubled.[1] Those higher fees all created higher premiums for the plans that had to pay them on behalf of the patients.

Having local control over some category of care is a persuasive, cost-expanding argument when there simply no longer is any "someplace else" to get that type of care. Plans and insurers need dermatology. They need cardiology. They need gastroenterology. They need many other specialty services. So when those horizontal specialty service consolidations happen, it's "game, set, and match" for the provider. Generally, the new prices have to be paid to the merged specialists, and premiums go up.

Monopoly Laws Are Hard to Apply to Local Markets

You might ask why that level of anticompetitive behavior doesn't trigger an antitrust investigation. There are two simple reasons. The first is that antitrust laws usually do not get invoked in these particular settings because the scope of the problem is too small and too local. When the federal government is focusing its legal teams on fighting Microsoft, it doesn't have time to look at hospital consolidation in Salt Lake City or Milwaukee or cardiology consolidation in any large U.S. city.

The second reason is that antitrust laws have a major flaw when it comes to health care. Anyone putting together a local health care merger can generally avoid running afoul of antitrust laws by proving that an alternate source of supply for that specific provider treatment exists and is "reasonably" accessible. Since health care monopolies tend to be very local, the providers that merge simply say, "There's another hospital only thirty miles away. People could go there. That proves we're not a monopoly." Under antitrust laws, the existence of the hospital thirty miles away does, in fact, make it hard to argue that the three closer hospitals have formed a monopoly by merging.

In the real world, however, patients don't like to drive past any local hospital to go thirty miles for care. They *could*, of course, do that, so the antitrust laws don't apply. They won't, however, join a health plan that forces them to make that thirty-mile drive, so real-world market forces both apply and prevail.

Health plans, of course, can't afford to have a thirty-mile hole in their provider map, so the formation of any solid single-specialty local monopoly is usually sufficient to jack prices up without triggering most federal and state antitrust laws. Care is amazingly local. Having all of the cardiology groups in a given hospital consolidate into one group is generally sufficient leverage to extract higher prices for heart care at that site. People don't want to drive (or be driven) very far when they are having a heart attack.

Across the country, provider mergers are continuing, and higher prices are the result. Boston hospitals have just received price increases from Boston health plans. Premium increases will quickly follow. San Diego hospitals recently canceled nearly ten dozen health plan contracts, telling plans to come back when they are ready to pay full fees. Most plans are paying. Premium hikes will follow.

Plan Negotiating Approaches Triggered the Provider Mergers

An objective observer might note that the plans brought this new provider development on themselves by being so aggressive in their demands for fee discounts. This is probably true.

The provider fee discounts of the 1990s truly did cut deep. The providers clearly had to respond. The new provider mergers are a perfectly understandable economic counterattack by the providers against the consolidated purchasing power of the plans. In many cases, the plan discounts were so low that they were unfair to the caregiver. It was hard for many hospitals and physician groups to stay in business while collecting about 60 percent of their fees.

Most provider mergers are not a proactive, long-term, deeply de-sired strategic attempt at achieving market control. They are, more often than not, mergers in self-defense. Most providers would prob-ably prefer never to merge.

That is particularly true of physician groups. Giving up inde-pendence is hard, and so is merging. Mergers are a real pain, and everyone now knows that. Nevertheless, done well, some mergers do work economically—but only when they create pricing power and negotiating leverage that can't happen as the result of any other strategy. Follow the money.

Successful mergers, once done, however, are hard to unravel. One Minnesota system has closed six of ten merged hospitals, markedly eliminating real competition from a major geographical area. That system has turned what had been a buyers' market for hospital care into a sellers' market. Those closed hospitals will be torn down or converted to other uses—senior housing, schools, or shopping malls. Most conversions of that sort are extremely hard to undo. Once hos-pitals are closed and converted to other uses, the unraveling is much less likely to occur. The country will feel those cost impacts for years to come, and the answer won't be to reopen old hospitals.

The long-term consequences of this merger and countless oth-ers like it across the country are huge: major increases in price, total loss of competitive provider forces, and a potentially permanent restructuring of local health care delivery.

If You Won't Buy "Curomyosin," You Can't Have "Fixomyacin"

On an even larger scale, the pharmaceutical companies have also gone through consolidations. Over the past dozen years, thirteen of the top twenty drug companies have merged with other pharmaceutical companies. Some of the new pharmaceutical giants—Pfizer, GlaxoSmithKline, and Bristol-Myers Squibb—are among the largest multinational companies in the world.[2]

Those drug company mergers fit the classical merger mode in very obvious ways, in some cases creating major market leverages for particular types of drugs. Some pharmaceutical companies have used the mergers to create drug packages for sale to health plans. Most health plans use drug formularies to improve care and cut costs; that is, they use teams of physicians and pharmacologists to select the best drugs for any given condition and negotiate a best price for the selected drugs (this subject is discussed in more detail in Chapter Six). The plans then ask participating physicians to use the formulary drugs for their patients. Premium savings usually result.

Generally, patient care is better as well, because the HMO formulary committees exclude specific drugs that don't work or work at minimal levels from the HMO formularies. A large percentage of commercially sold drugs are, in fact, class C drugs—drugs that do not outperform other available drugs but are allowed on the market by the U.S. Food and Drug Administration (FDA) merely because they outperformed a placebo in clinical trials. Those less effective drugs tend not to be included in HMO formularies because HMOs can't afford to use drugs that don't work.

In that formulary development process, some highly profitable but less useful drugs are eliminated from the list of drugs used by plan doctors. The drug companies hate those formularies. They would like to keep selling all of the profitable and less effective drugs that were rejected by the pharmaceutical review committees. So some megacompanies now use their new leverage to say, "You love 'Curomysin' for arthritis, but you won't use our 'Fixomycin' for toe fungus. Guess what? If you don't include 'Fixomycin' on your formulary, we won't give you a decent price on 'Curomycin.' Your costs will go way up. Your doctors will be angry. It's a package deal. We now own both drugs. Take both or you get none. You decide." This process has brought some less useful drugs back into many HMO formularies and further increased the annual costs of care.

The drug company mergers have also allowed some megacompanies to gain control over major producers of generic drugs. There is no reason to believe that approach will result in lower prices for the generic drugs. The megapharmacy companies are also almost impossible to unravel. No one will cut them up and make them compete with each other again.

A major problem for the pharmaceutical industry today is a shortage of new drugs projected for release three to five years from now. It can be assumed that excessive consolidation is resulting in more rigid controls on research agendas, resulting in less creativity and therefore fewer useful new chemicals. From a quality-of-care perspective, that isn't a good thing.

Physician Cartels Will Make the Price Situation Worse

To the amazement of anyone concerned about health care costs, Congress has recently been wrestling with the possibility of creating new antitrust exemption laws that will make it easier for physicians in various markets to band together into local pricing cartels. The goal is to create much greater contracting leverage for the doctors. To gain support from the more liberal members of the government, lobbyists for the physicians refer to the cartels (very cleverly and disingenuously) as "physician unions." Don't look for those "unions" to qualify for membership in the AFL-CIO anytime soon. Also, don't look to them as a mechanism to stabilize or reduce costs. Pure mergers in many markets have caused fees to jump anywhere from 10 to 150 percent. Cartels should create the same range of major fee increases without the providers' having to go through the whole merger process.

Since health insurance premiums are simply the arithmetic sum of the cost of care, the fee increases caused by these doctor cartels will be passed on directly to consumers, dollar for dollar, through premium increases.

Legislators who vote for those cartels should start early explaining to local voters why increasing both unit fees and provider procedure prices are good economics for consumers. It's very likely that health plans will now begin to publicize the cartel-based price increases. Plans have finally learned not to keep that information silent.

In any case, providers everywhere are now vigorously counterattacking against a decade of market division and HMO-imposed price constraints. As providers win in various markets, costs go up. As providers win in multiple markets, premiums explode. These trends won't abate soon.

6

. . . .

Does the United States Pay Fair
Prices by World Standards?

How do care prices in the United States compare to the rest of the world?

It's obvious to any observer of international health care that our physicians, nurses, and other caregivers make more money than their counterparts in any other country. Doctors from all over the world emigrate to the United States in large part because the pay scale for physicians in this country eclipses world standards. Most doctors in Santiago, Chile, make less than $35,000 a year. Most doctors in Moscow make even less. Doctors in Canada and Great Britain are lucky to make $100,000 a year. The average pay in America is $144,000 for primary care physicians and $246,000 for specialists.[1]

Likewise, the cost for a day in the hospital in the United States far exceeds the cost of a hospital day in Canada or Great Britain.[2]

These higher costs contribute to making ours the most expensive health care infrastructure in the world. Our baseline expenses are far higher than in any other country. In almost every area of care, our costs are higher than world averages and are going up.

It's a good thing that we don't have to sell routine front-line health care services in the context of a world market. If we did, our prices would be significantly out of line with the rest of the planet.

But it's actually not that hard to justify our high costs for hospital and medical care. We have exceptional hospitals and wonderful physicians in the United States. Anyone who has traveled in other countries and visited their hospitals, as we have, can tell you that the facilities, equipment, technology, and care standards in the United States are a full cut above all but a very few premier hospitals in other countries. Most hospitals in other countries are underfunded, understaffed, old, and very crowded. They tend to be highly underequipped. Regulators would close most of those hospitals almost immediately if they were located in any state in the United States.

Our physicians are likewise well trained and generally highly competent. New U.S. physicians have little trouble passing international licensing exams. Medical school graduates from many other countries have appalling large failure rates on these same exams. U.S. physicians are paid well, but in the context of a society that pays other professions equally well. The total take-home pay of U.S. physicians accounts for less than 20 percent of our total health care costs, so those direct payments are not the primary factor that differentiates us from the rest of the world in costs.

The whole issue of provider consolidation and pricing trends is dealt with later in this book. Some of those trends are beginning to have a real upward pressure on U.S. health care expenses. A defender of those trends might point out that they also should be reviewed in the context of local economic conditions and not judged against world standards.

Drug Costs in the United States Are Substantially Higher Than in Other Nations

One area where U.S. health care prices can be compared very directly to the rest of the world is relative to prescription drugs. Prilosec in the United States is exactly the same drug as Prilosec in Canada or Tasmania.

So how do we stack up on our expenses and costs for these identical chemical products? And how are we doing on U.S. drug prices from year to year?

Take a look first at relative drug prices. Drug prices in this country are now increasing by 15 to 20 percent each year. And the fact is that drugs overall get better and better. What are we getting for that money? Let's look at a few drugs.

No one argues that Claritin and Allegra are superior drugs for many people with seasonal allergic rhinitis or that Prilosec and Aciphex are great drugs for esophageal reflux. No one denies that Imitrex can help keep many people from the deep misery of a migraine. Each of those drugs helps make lives better. Americans use them all the time.

But do Americans pay fair prices for those drugs? A month's supply of Prilosec, for example, costs $99.95 in the United States. That same quantity, made by the same manufacturer, costs $50.88 in Canada. It costs even less in Mexico: $17.50.[3] Thirty pills of Prevacid cost $127.49 at a Minnesota drugstore and $41.89 if you buy them over the Internet from Canada.[4] (It's against the law to buy them over the Internet, but if you did, you'd eliminate more than two-thirds of the cost.) Imitrex costs $30.00 in the United States, $11 in Mexico, and $9.20 in Canada.

Cross the American border into Mexico, and what is the first thing you see? Drugstores selling prescription drugs to American patients, often at 25 cents on the dollar.

When the antihistamine Claritin was a prescription drug, a month's supply of it, for example, cost about $80 in the United States, compared to $10 to $15 in dozens of other countries where it is sold over the counter.[5] Claritin is now being sold over the counter in the United States for about $30 for a month's supply.

Medical technology prices also vary tremendously between the United States and other countries. Heart stents, for example, cost $1,200 to $1,400 each in the United States and $400 in Canada. Laser eye surgery costs roughly between $1,200 and $2,000 in the United States. That same surgery costs between and $400 and $600 in Canada. Similar examples abound.

Why do suppliers of drugs and technology charge so much more in the United States than they do in Canada, Japan, or Peru? Because they can. And, ironically, because they can, they must. This is an important fact for Americans to understand.

What would happen to the president of a multinational publicly held drug firm who announced to her stockholders, "We are now charging unfairly high prices in the United States! So starting Monday, I am going to bring our U.S. prices down 50 percent to align them with the prices we charge in Europe. Of course, those particular American price cuts will reduce our overall corporate profits for next year by 80 percent because we currently make most of our profits in the United States. It's entirely possible, as a result, that the profit cuts will reduce the market value of your stocks in our company. The stock you own could be worth a bit less—maybe even a lot less. But, hey, get over it. Fairness isn't easy, but it's just plain fair."

How long would that drug company CEO keep her job? Minutes at best. Stockholders would rise up to fire the board if the board didn't quickly fire the president. Class action suits could result, with angry stockholders accusing management of incompetence.

"Fairness" is not a market standard for drug prices that will carry much weight in corporate boardrooms if that pricing fairness results in pharmaceutical company stock price collapse and executive firings.

How did the United States get into this mess in the first place? Why are U.S. drug and technology prices so much higher than elsewhere?

Market Forces Are Neutered in the United States for Prescription Drugs

To understand both the recent massive increase in drug prices and overall U.S. drug pricing levels, it is important to step back to see the context in which American drug prices are created. In the United States, drug prices can be set at almost any level because, under many of today's insurance laws, consumers have a "right" to the use of any drug that works. That "right" is not limited by any of the normal market forces that apply to determining the value or purchase of most products in a free economy.

Ironically, although the United States supposedly has a market-driven health care economy (in contrast to the more monolithic, government-run health care systems of almost all other countries), basic and fundamental value-based market forces are blunted here. By contrast, in the government-managed health care economies, a form of buyer-seller value equation does function fairly well to help keep drug prices down.

How can that be true? Think about how the various national government-run systems relate value to price. For example, if a drug company wants to sell a new arthritis drug, how does that drug get priced and sold in countries that have a single-payer, government-run health insurance model?

In nations with a fixed national health budget, the drug companies must negotiate a price directly with the government. "We'd like two dollars a pill," the manufacturer's salesperson might tell the minister of health.

"What good does the drug do?" the minister might ask.

"Well, it reduces arthritis inflammation."

"Fine," the minister might say. "How much better is it than the old inflammation reduction drug we have now that costs us ten cents a pill?"

"Well," the manufacturer might reply, "our tests show the new drug reduces pain 5 percent better than your current drug."

At that point, classical market forces come into play. Value becomes relevant. Is a 5 percent improvement in pain relief worth a 2,000 percent increase in price?

"Sorry," the minister might say. "Two dollars a pill isn't a good deal. We'll just keep using the old drug."

"Well," the pharmaceutical representative might reply. "Let's not be hasty. Two dollars is just our American retail price. We can do better. How about fifty cents a pill? Would you buy them for your patients for fifty cents?"

"No," the health minister says. "You're still increasing our costs 500 percent for only a 5 percent improvement in care. That, my friend, is not a good deal for our taxpayers."

The value judgment that must be made at that point about the cost benefit of the drug becomes a real challenge for the minister of health. Pain relief is good. People want pain relief. Voters want pain relief. But how much relief at what price? Typically, after some dickering between the manufacturer and the minister, a value-based price is agreed on. If the 5 percent increase in care value is not significant enough to justify spending more money, that particular new drug may never be sold in that country. Market forces keep it out. What market forces? A decision by the actual payer (the government) that the price of the drug exceeds its perceived value.

More likely, the drug company will say, "Okay, your excellency, we'll give the drug to you for 25 cents a pill, but not a farthing less." And a deal is done.

By contrast, look at how that same drug manufacturer would set a price when that same drug is introduced into the United States. The American steps are simple. First, the drug manufacturer would arbitrarily set a price, a highly profitable price. Then the manufacturer would run ads in various consumer and medical magazines touting the drug. For some drugs, TV, radio, and newspaper ads would be run. In addition, the manufacturer would send an army of highly trained salespeople into the field to call directly on all relevant doctors. The salespeople would urge each individual doctor to "try" the drug. In some cases, physicians have been given various kinds of gifts to help persuade them to prescribe particular drugs.

The advertising copy that would run in *Time* magazine or a similar publication might say something like this: "*Pain Away*—proven in clinical tests to measurably outperform every other available pain-killing drug for arthritis. Ask your doctor to prescribe it for you. Pain hurts. We can help. We're on your side. Pain Away. You need it."

We've all seen similar ads like this. They often promise miracles, or near miracles.

The actual, and minor, 5 percent pain level improvement statistic would not typically show up in the drug company ad, and certainly not as 5 percent. The typical reference would be that it is "measurably" better. Nor would the ad mention the price. It certainly wouldn't be featured. Consumers who see the ads would be led to think, *This drug will save me a lot of pain, and it won't cost me any more than my current drug because all I ever pay out of my own pocket is the insurance copay anyway.*

Studies show that the vast majority of doctors who find themselves facing patients carrying those ads simply give in to the patient and prescribe whatever expensive chemical the ad is pushing as long as the patients actually have the disease that the drug is said to treat.[6]

Large-volume purchasers in this country like HMOs and some huge prescription drug administrators generally manage to negotiate meaningful discounts off the drug company's standard retail price. That negotiated lower price for the drug saves premium money for HMO patients because premiums are, of course, the "arithmetic sum of the cost of care." But those negotiated discounts in the United States seldom, if ever, are anywhere near as low as Canadian retail prices.

Is Advertising the Best Way to Promote Drugs?

In the United States, the drug companies work very intelligently to create direct consumer demand for highly profitable drugs as quickly as possible. They often advertise the drugs directly to consumers through multiple media outlets. They spend billions of dollars on consumer advertising: $2.5 billion in 2000, a 35 percent increase over 1999.[7] About 30 percent[8] of total pharmaceutical company budgets are now spent on marketing drugs and administration compared to roughly 20 percent[9] spent on researching new drugs.

Prilosec alone was the beneficiary of $79.4 million dollars worth of advertising in 1999. Claritin received $137.1 million in direct-to-consumer advertising that same year. Sales for Prilosec went up 23.9 percent. Claritin sales went up 21.1 percent. Advertising clearly works.

To be fair, the ads can do some good in encouraging people to seek care for their medical condition. A 1998 *Prevention* magazine study reported that direct-to-consumer advertising resulted in more than 21 million people talking with their doctors about a medical condition or illness for the first time.[10] That's good news. It's a step forward for each of those people. It's also expensive news, in the short term, because it means that 21 million more people are receiving care. If you believe that treating disease early is good (and we do), then there is a good result for the whole process. But increasing consumers' interest in care through advertising is one more factor to understand as we look at why health care costs are rising so rapidly right now.

The way we pay for drugs in this country does create some real problems in drug use. Value, as a science-based, objectively measured decision factor, is too often not part of doctors' and consumers' decision process in that typical American ad-based drug distribution system. Consumers see ads and demand drugs, and, more often than not, doctors write the prescriptions—whether or not those drugs actually add much value.

Are consumers discerning, value-based buyers when it comes to drugs? Look at the recent flu drug, which was heavily advertised in 2001. The ads made it sound as if the flu drug offered incredible benefits. They claimed their drug "attacks the influenza virus and stops it from spreading inside your body. It treats flu at its source, by attacking the virus that causes the flu rather than simply masking symptoms." Those are persuasive words, and they created market demand.

The drug costs about $53 per episode, about four times the price of over-the-counter drugs or the flu shot.[11] Still, doesn't it sound like a good deal? Who wouldn't spend $53 to avoid the flu? There was just one problem: The drug didn't work quite as well as the ads might imply. Data on the actual efficacy did exist, but they were not built into the ad campaign. Why? Because on average, tests showed that the drug actually reduced the duration of a flu episode by about one day.[12]

That's a benefit, but how much of a benefit? Would a minister of health of some value-based purchasing country, working with a tight health care budget, pay more than fifty dollars per patient for a new drug whose real value was basically to reduce a multiday case of the flu by about one day? The minister might for people in needed industries or for military people on standby. But on balance, the typical minister of health would probably prefer to spend his or her country's finite health budget on another drug or procedure that offered more value to more people.

In the United States, many thousands of flu victims saw the ads. They then demanded—and received—that drug. More often than not, the drug was paid for by their health plan. Or to be more ac-curate, it was paid for in everyone's monthly premiums.

Lyme disease vaccine comes to mind as another heavily adver-tised drug that might well have trouble passing a rigorous minister of health value screen. Extensive and somewhat frightening TV ads recently told urban Americans that Lyme disease could strike in the heart of the biggest city. A great many Americans asked for and re-ceived those shots.

What facts would a minister of health consider? The vaccine costs $180 per patient.[13] One study indicated that less than one case of Lyme disease per 100,000 occurs in urban areas.[14] If that were true, the minister would need to vaccinate 100,000 city dwellers at a total cost of $18 million to prevent one case of the disease.

Is that sufficient value? Lyme can be a debilitating disease. In Minnesota, HealthPartners is studying the use of the Lyme vaccine drug right now. Who should get it? What value does it offer? Are some people much more likely to be exposed?

Interestingly, there's more to the story than just the cost per case. Any competent minister of health worth holding the job would also recognize that once people receive that vaccine, any further diagnostic tests done by a physician to determine whether an individual actually has the disease becomes highly inaccurate—problematic at best. Subsequent cases of Lyme disease could go undiagnosed.

If everyone were vaccinated, some actual cases of the disease might be overlooked. Furthermore, many people who did have the disease could be overtreated due to false-positive readings on Lyme disease tests. In other words, a reasonable evaluation would look at the total impact of widespread use of vaccine.

These are not necessarily good outcomes for those particular directly affected people.

Think of these issues when you see the next Lyme disease ads. Used appropriately, the vaccine can add value. In an area with a high incidence of the disease, it might save a lot of suffering and costs. The overall issue is not an easy one to call. The drug company's position is clear. The ads are clear. All other parties have a more complex set of factors to consider.

In any case, the ads work: people ask for the drug, many get it, and everyone's premiums go up.

The public needs to understand too the fact that some of the new blockbuster drugs are no more effective than the medications they replace and are much more expensive.

When it was a prescription drug, Claritin, the most profitable antihistamine of all time, cost around $80 in the United States compared to such inexpensive over-the-counter drugs as Chlor-Trimeton, Benadryl, and Tavist.[15] Many of these new drugs have roughly equivalent effects on allergic symptoms but vary in the number of pills that need to be taken per day and sedating side effects. What value should be assigned to these benefits? What cost? Who should pay it?

The problems that result from both overpricing and excessive advertising of prescription drugs in the United States are open to debate. As this book was being written, federal legislators were discussing a proposed bill that could provide greater oversight of direct-to-consumer drug advertising.[16] And the U.S. Food and Drug Administration is reexamining its 1997 decision to loosen requirements for broadcast ads. These discussions are the result of government concern about ads' contributing to the rising costs of prescription drugs.[17] Those same issues apply to the use of medical technology.

Drug costs are a major problem for America's senior citizens. Most Medicare patients have no coverage for prescription drugs, a real problem because no one needs prescription drugs more than seniors do. Chronic care patients can easily run up drug bills of hundreds of dollars each month. When these costs exceed the patient's ability to pay, the care is compromised and lives are damaged. That issue needs to be resolved.

Drug costs now create a major problem for the population under age sixty-five as well. For the first time in history, prescription drug costs have exceeded hospital care costs for a small but growing number of employer groups. Two decades ago, hospital costs were roughly 50 percent of total health care cost expenditures.[18] Drug costs in that era were 5.5 percent of total costs.[19] Today, inpatient hospital costs are down to under 30 percent of the total (up in actual dollars but down as a percentage). Drug costs have climbed in both dollars and percentages (12 to 14 percent), to the point where, for a small number of older employer groups, health plans now spend more money on drug claims than hospital claims.

Between 1995 and 1999, drug expenditures in the United States more than doubled, from $65 billion to $125 billion. One government study projects that drug spending in this country will nearly double again by 2008, reaching $243 billion.[20]

Some medical experts claim that the new drugs, in total, will ultimately save money because they can reduce or eliminate hospital stays for many patients. For some individual patients, that is definitely true. That point is yet to be proven for entire patient populations, however. It may well turn out to be accurate. It deserves careful actuarial review, but it's a speculative claim at best today.

We hope it turns out to be true. So do the drug companies.

Formularies Pushed the Worst
Drugs out of the Market

In any case, we do know that drugs are getting better every day. HMOs and other health plans should get some of the credit for that improvement.

Why? Because two decades ago, 84 percent of drugs brought to market were class C drugs—only better than a placebo.[21] Many drugs were brought to market more for their ability to generate sales than for their ability to cure a disease. HMOs changed that practice by instituting drug formularies. HMOs created committees of pharmacologists and physicians to figure out which drugs actually worked for any given health condition. Hundreds of class C drugs were cut from the HMOs' approved list of drugs. Then the HMOs negotiated with the drug companies for discounts on the drugs that actually worked. Once the discounts were in place, the plans urged their doctors to use those drugs.

The good news in that process was that the plans stopped using hundreds of less useful drugs. Even better news was the drug companies' realization that developing new batches of class C drugs was no longer a profitable strategy. Once HMOs started screening drugs to figure out which ones actually worked, the drug companies' best strategy was to develop drugs that worked better so that the HMOs would be forced to select those drugs for their formularies. That new dynamic changed the focus of the pharmaceutical marketplace. All Americans benefited from that new focus on drugs that actually work.

The pharmaceutical companies also refocused on drugs for chronic care patients, developing drugs that patients would be taking for the rest of their lives. Patients benefited because the new drugs made their lives better. Drug companies benefited because sales went up, as did prices.

Do we pay fair prices for drugs in the United States? Probably not. We can't afford to be the funder for all drug research in the world, while other counties pay for their drugs based only on the cost of production, not development. All payers should share the costs of development.

To be fair, a strong argument can be made that without the huge revenue subsidy and incentives that are embedded in U.S. drug prices, the pharmaceutical companies would need to cut back on their research. If their revenues shrink, their product development dollars will shrink as well. If that happens, we'll see a slowing in the pace of new drugs and new medical tools. The momentum of miracles will decrease. Miracles cost money. We need to figure out what trade-offs we are willing to make.

Overall, with prescription drugs, medical procedures, and medical technology, no one can dispute the fact that the care levels of 2003 are far better than the care levels of 1993. No one with any serious disease would want to substitute 1993 care for today's care.

We do miracles today. The only downside is that those miracles cost money. Sometimes they cost more money here than they do elsewhere in the world.

How the Internet Is Changing Health Care

I Learned About My Prosthesis on the Web

The Internet has become a major cost factor in health care. Because of the Internet, patients are better informed, more demanding, and have higher expectations for their care. The volumes of Internet use are immense: almost 100 million adult Americans now use the Internet for health care information.[1] Some Internet experts believe that more people now use the Net for health information than for shopping or pornography.

Across the country, doctors report that when they tell a patient that he or she has a serious disease, more often than not, the patient goes home, cranks up a favorite Web search engine, and looks up the condition. Huge amounts of data about treatments, symptoms, and diagnosis are available—some good, some not good at all. If the patient doesn't personally look up the condition on the Web, then a child, spouse, niece, nephew, cousin, grandchild, coworker, or neighbor generally will do it for him or her.

Then when the patient reenters the doctor's office for that first postdiagnosis visit, the scenario is very different from what it would have been only two or three years ago. Back then, a patient with a dread disease or complex condition came to the doctor's office humbly hoping that the all-knowing and hopefully all-powerful physician could explain the medical condition and plot out a cure. The doctor was the sole source of relevant knowledge and, in almost all cases, the sole source of medical strategy.

The physician would define the condition and then tell the patient what the preferred treatment "should" be. Patients would tell their friends, "Dr. Jones says I should be operated on next week. Boy, I'm sure glad I have her for a doctor." The doctor's words, in that pre-Web interaction, were gold.

Today, thanks to the Internet, the patient often returns to the exam room bearing an armful of Internet printouts and remarkably well informed about the disease and eager to discuss care alternatives. That's a revolutionary change in the caregiver-patient relationship. It is incredibly empowering for the patient. Medical issues are no longer purely medical mysteries resolved only by all-powerful, all-knowing medical gurus. Physicians are still highly respected and powerful gurus, but they are no longer the only gurus in the game.

So why is that particular phenomenon relevant to a book about health care costs? Because patient expectations about the nature, extent, and scope of care are changing, and these expectations are also proving expensive. Better-informed patients are more demanding. Patients no longer passively accept whatever treatments their physicians recommend. Instead, they increasingly feel as if they are partners in their own care, able to understand care alternatives and express preferences.

As a side note, this change in roles has been a difficult adjustment for many older physicians. Some do not like feeling challenged by patients. One well-known doctor in Minnesota told patients, "If you're going to get your diagnosis and treatment information on the Web, get your care off the Web too. Get out of my office. Go to the Web doctor for your care."

Fortunately, that perspective isn't held by many physicians. Some of the best and most enlightened medical schools are beginning to teach students how to use the new wealth of Web research done by patients as a useful and convenient extension of the doctors' own research efforts. Those schools teach the new physicians how to sort quickly through the patient's armload of Web printouts to find the ones that originate from credible sources and might contain useful information.

Most medical school students today come from the computer generation. They not only are comfortable with Web-based information; they expect it. It's hard to convince a student who has done research on the Web through high school and college to learn to use classical paper textbooks at medical school.

Web Sites Can Improve Care

This new Web involvement in care has two very different impacts on costs. On the one hand, the Web creates demanding patients. On the other hand, the Web has the potential to enhance the effectiveness of physicians.

Knowledgeable patients are quite often more demanding patients. Some medical conditions are relatively rare. Physicians may see them only infrequently, if at all. Conditions such as muscular dystrophy, cancer of the rectum, gout, and chronic renal failure tend to be less than 1 percent of a given primary care doctor's practice.[2] In other words, many doctors have traditionally treated relatively infrequently seen conditions even though those conditions are not part of the doctor's daily patient load and even though each doctor's personal knowledge about the most effective and successful current practices for these rare diseases may not be entirely up to date.

Some doctors do a magnificent job of caring for those patients. Others do less well. No one knows which doctors do what. What we do know is that treatments for those conditions vary widely from town to town, practice to practice, and doctor to doctor. In one study, 135 doctors who were all given the same patient example came up with eighty-two different treatments.[3]

A Given Condition May Be 1 Percent of a Doctor's Practice but 100 Percent of a Patient's Care

Patients start out with a very limited overall array of medical knowledge. That now often changes when patients learn that they have an alarming diagnosis. For the most part, patients with a serious medical issue quickly begin to seek information about their condition. That makes obvious sense. From the patient's perspective, the statistical ratios relative to the frequency of the disease work in direct contrast to the physician's ratios. In other words, a given medical condition may make up only one-half of 1 percent of a given physician's practice, but for a patient who suffers personally from that particular condition, that diagnosis represents 100 percent of the patient's medical status. That personal focus gives the patient a huge incentive to become at least a lay expert on that one disease.

As patients become Web-trained "experts," quite often they start suggesting care options to the doctor. Those care options may involve expensive drugs, expensive specialty referrals, or expensive medical procedures. Patients sometimes know where the best new research on their disease is being done before their doctors even know that the new research exists.

For the most part, the result is better care. It never hurts any physician to get the most current medical information about a given condition. Web printouts can help.

Web Sites Can Also Lead to Bad Care

Unfortunately, however, not all information on the Web is accurate. Some is glaringly, even dangerously, inaccurate. That can create real problems, particularly when the Web sites seem credible to the patient. There are no standards for inclusion on the Internet. Anyone can offer health advice on the Web. There's no screening process for determining who is an appropriately trained and licensed source of Web information and who is a crackpot. Reeducating misled patients can and does waste a lot of doctors' valuable energy and time, adding to the cost of care.

Another Web issue relates back to that persistent problem area of "unproven" care. Complications arise between patients and doctors and patients and plans when the care suggestions that the patient found on the Internet involve untried, unproven, currently experimental care. Recall that most experimental care isn't covered by insurance. Some highly subjective Web sites can make various kinds of untested care sound wonderful and successful beyond belief. Anecdotes abound, and in most of those anecdotes, miracles happen. Those anecdotes don't have to be accurate to be influential; they just need to be available. The Web makes them available.

Patients with serious illnesses who learn about supposedly promising experimental programs in distant medical research centers can sometimes put huge pressure on their local doctor to refer them to such centers. These patients can also put pressure on their health plan to pay for the care if they are treated in such centers. In those sad instances where the patient's prognosis is extremely poor with standard treatment and the research is being done by credible scientists, there is often a powerful and totally logical pressure exerted by patients who believe those programs give them their only chance of success—maybe their only chance of living. When that happens, all of the experimental care issues discussed in Chapter Three are activated.

Another Web-generated problem is patients' demanding nontraditional care that is entirely outside the bounds of normal insurance coverage. A huge number of Web sites offer opinions and information about nontraditional care: aromatherapy comes to mind, or energy therapy for breast cancer, or music therapy for anxiety. Many Web sites are flush with anecdotal testimonials about the supposed efficacy of the alternative care.

Because most traditional physicians don't make referrals to those kinds of non-science-based caregivers and because most health plans do not pay for those kinds of services, this is another area where the Web is having a stressful, cost-expanding impact on traditional care.

Some of the most significant cost pressures are due to the Web sites of various condition-specific advocacy groups. These sites often strongly recommend care approaches not covered by traditional insurance. Parents of autistic children, for example, offer several Web sites that feature untraditional, unproven, experimental care approaches. These approaches generally cannot be covered by insurance until they are proven to work by a formal research process. Understandably, loving, and sometimes desperate, parents do not want to wait for the completion of a formal research process, particularly when some other parents may already be claiming on the Web that the experimental or nonstandard treatment definitely worked for their own kids. These Web sites clearly create cost pressures on care and create conflicts between patients and doctors and patients and payers.

Again, it's absolutely easy to understand the patient's perspective. If a person is dying of cancer or some other dread disease and has been told by the doctor that death is inevitable, then any care alternative that seems to promise even a 1 percent chance of survival can look pretty good.

Most people are not actuaries or mathematicians. A 1 percent chance of survival becomes translated and reinterpreted in the minds of most people to actually mean "chance versus no chance" or "choice versus no choice," or, in a nutshell, "hope versus no hope."

That yes/no, hope/no hope context feels emotionally like fifty-fifty or even 100 percent (a chance) versus zero (no chance). People want a chance. They want a chance to live. They want a chance for their child to walk or talk. One percent is an important, context-setting, and numerically weighted decision factor for a mathematician. It's the only hope for the parent of a dying child.

As those payout patterns grow and experimental care becomes a more common expense for health plans, insurers, and various government programs, we can expect a further increase in the rate of health care cost growth. Many of those experiments can be extremely expensive. One experimental program for autistic children was priced at $500,000 per child. That might be a reasonable price if the program had been proven in vigorous clinical trials to work. It's a lot of money to pay for an unproven experiment. But because it was featured on a Web site, it created a lot of pressure with some understandably frustrated parents of autistic children.

In 2000, the United States spent nearly $4.5 billion on various kinds of clinical trials. More than 80 percent of this spending came from biotechnology, medical device, and pharmaceutical companies.[4] If the trend continues, the amount of money spent on clinical trials and experimental care will continue to climb, keeping the rate of increase in research costs at an all-time-high level.

As each new procedure, technology, and treatment is shown to work, that information will be widely communicated over the Internet, and patient expectations will continue to work in favor of ever more expensive care. The American philosophy of health is, "When it works, we use it—and insurance pays for it." That philosophy is strongly supported by the existence of the Web.

An even more exciting use of the Web relates to having a wide array of scientific knowledge and data about medical best practices available to the actual physician or other caregivers. Physicians traditionally have had to hunt down their own scientific updates through what is often a relatively haphazard process that includes seminars, journal articles, and salespeople from drug companies and medical equipment manufacturers. We are now moving beyond that point to having search engines for physicians that can do a much more thorough, complete, and timely review of the available source and literature for individual patients. In the very best settings, that information is available to the physician on a computer screen in the exam room, as well as being available for more complete review later in the privacy of the physician's office.

The best systems not only bring that information to the physician. They also create instant printouts for patients showing the exact nature of their disease and the appropriate next steps for dealing with it.

That topic is covered in more detail later in the context of automated medical records and supportive systems of care. Architects, engineers, lawyers, and other professionals already use comparable computer support technology. It's almost ready for use by physicians.

Care will definitely improve and become more consistent when those tools are in place.

Net Care, e-Care, More Care

The Internet is more than a library. It can also be used to deliver care. The use of the Net for care delivery will grow dramatically over the next several years. Direct Net consultations from medical experts will become common. Perhaps a third of current office visits will become unnecessary, replaced by far more convenient Web contacts. House calls, that is, virtual house calls, will return for a great many patients. Visual linkages will enable doctors to see patients in their homes, and technology in the home will be able to provide weight, pulse, temperature, and blood pressure information and even, for selected patients with specific diseases, blood chemistry and selected lab test reports.

How will these developments affect the cost of care?

Done well, they could both improve care and reduce the costs of care. They should, at a minimum, significantly improve patient access to certain kinds of care. Web cams will allow for middle-of-the-night "face-to-face" consultations that would otherwise require inconvenient and even wasteful trips to urgent care or emergency settings. Follow-up care is particularly amenable to Web interactions.

There is, however, a major obstacle in place right now to Web-based medicine: providers won't do it if they can't get paid for it. Right now, most insurers do not pay for Web-based care. Insurers need to learn how to pay for those types of services. Some form of charge structure has to be created. Most Web care now is not reimbursed by insurers, self-insured employers, or government programs. Why not? In part, because of the fear that costs will explode if Web-based care is available. Some payers are afraid that greedy revenue-seeking providers might decide, for example, that their chronic care patients all need two or three billable extra "Web consults" a week rather than one billable face-to-face consult every two weeks.

Payers worry that patients will find Web access to their own doc-tor so convenient and even pleasant that they will seek Web care constantly for very minor care issues. Hypochondriacs could find access to their physician only two Web clicks away. Every day. Likewise, some people just like attention, especially caregiver attention.

The problem could be a particular challenge for Medicare patients. For seniors with transportation problems, Web-based interaction with their caregivers could be a real blessing. But contact might become too easy. How many Medicare patients will take advantage of the opportunity to discuss their health issues daily? How many lonely older folks will use the Web and their doctor as a way of having contact with someone who cares? What will all of that contact cost?

Who will set standards for that care? Who will set unit prices? Who will know when the payment system is being abused to generate excess profits?

These issues have to be resolved soon. Many medical practices are currently refusing to do Web care for their patients because the care is not billable at any level. Patients now want it, but providers can't survive economically if a large portion of their formerly billable in-office care is suddenly delivered on the Web free of charge. It's hard for a medical group to meet payroll if too much care becomes free.

Patients want Web care now. Web care and e-visits both make immense sense. They can make care easier and more convenient for millions of patients. Those developments represent the next major service enhancement for care delivery. In multispecialty medical groups like the ones we work for, the uses of that tool are obvious and compelling. The challenge will be to resolve all of the relevant issues in a way that creates the best and most convenient care for patients while paying providers fairly for their time and expertise.

In health plans where the care system is exclusively part of the overall plan, many of the fee-for-service e-visit issues disappear. Plans like Group Health of Puget Sound, Kaiser Permanente, and HealthPartners will probably be pioneers in delivering care over the Net, in part because they work with salaried physicians, not just with fee-based physicians.

Long-Distance Care

Another nice feature of the Net is that it makes distances disappear. Web care can be done continents away. A patient who has a heart attack in Spain may be able—with the right system—to have his complete medical record sent in seconds from his U.S. doctor to his Spanish caregiver.

Long-distance care will soon become a way of having the best providers in America (Mayo Clinic) able to provide specialty consultations in other countries or even in other regions of this country. The good news is that that level of specialty service could restore competition for some services in certain otherwise monopolistic markets. The bad news is that local providers in many markets are seeking to use local licensing laws to prevent use of that level of Internet care.

In any case, the Web is transforming care. Up to this point, the primary impact has been to add expense. Over time, that impact may change. More consistent care may reduce the costly complications that result from less-than-optimal care. In either case, care has already improved. And "we ain't seen nothing yet."

8

The Coming Crunch in Health Care Workers

Ask any hospital administrator what his or her number one logistical problem will be for the next several years, and the odds are good that the response will be "staffing."

We already are facing a shortage of health care workers for a great many job classifications. Nurses, technicians, pharmacists, and other crucial members of the health care delivery team are in short supply in many areas. And the problem will get much worse before it gets better (see Figure 8.1). To keep existing workers and attract new ones, hospitals, clinics, and other care programs are all increasing wages for their care staff well beyond current wage increases in the rest of the economy.

These salary cost increases are added to the bill for each hospital and institutional care site. The higher bills result in higher premium needs for plans and insurers. At this point, it appears that we have both a short- and a long-range problem.

Who Will Empty My Bedpan and Monitor My Brain Scan?

Take a look at nursing. We have more jobs than nurses now, and the long-term trend lines are extremely discouraging. By the year 2020, projections are that there will be a shortage of 800,000 registered nurses (RNs).[1] From 2000 to 2006, demand for nursing jobs

Figure 8.1. Unfilled Job Rate in Selected Health Care Positions

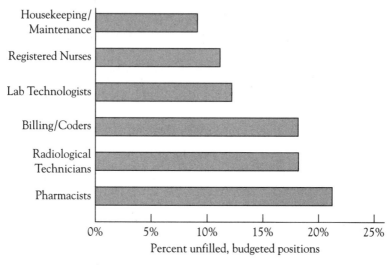

Source: American Hospital Association *TrendWatch*, June 2001, Vol. 3, No. 2.

is projected to grow by 23 percent, yet there has been a steep decline in enrollment in nursing schools—a decrease of 20.9 percent over that same period alone.[2] A recent study predicts a shortage of 168,000 nurses by 2006 if current graduation rates don't increase.[3] Since it takes four years to prepare a nurse, enrollments would have to increase immediately to meet that need. There is no sign that it is going to happen.

The shortage of nurses could mean the difference between life and death. A University of Pennsylvania study found that patients recovering from common surgeries at hospitals with fewer nurses per patient have a greater risk of dying. Researchers compared hospitals with varying nurse staffing ratios and calculated that if all hospitals nationally used the ratio with the fewest nurses per patient, the death rate would increase by 31 percent, or as many as twenty thousand avoidable deaths annually.[4]

Anecdotes about the nursing shortage abound. In Texas, Virginia, and California, the nursing shortage has forced some hospitals to close units and turn away patients. At one Los Angeles hospital, the nursing position vacancy rate is around 12 percent (100 unfilled jobs), and it can take up to six months to fill certain specialty nursing jobs.[5] This is not unusual today. The average vacancy rate for hospital nursing jobs across the country was 14.7 percent in 2000.[6]

In Baltimore's Johns Hopkins Hospital, needed surgical beds were recently idled because of a shortage of nurses, forcing delays in some elective surgeries. In Boston, Brigham and Women's Hospital closed 15 of its 650 beds for about eight weeks in the summer of 2000, in part because of the nursing shortage.[7] Those aren't huge reductions in capacity, but they are the beginning of a trend.

In Minnesota, a recent contract between RNs and local hospitals gave the nurses the right to close admissions to any hospital unit if the nurses believe that the unit is understaffed. The understaffing is the result of hospitals' not being able to hire enough nurses. Prior to the new contract, the hospitals would fill the beds with patients and ask the nurses to work overtime. In the new arrangement, those patients will need to find another hospital or another unit within the hospital.

In New York City, it now takes from six to nine months to fill certain specialized nursing jobs, such as operating room and labor and delivery nurses.[8]

A Vermont study stated in January 2000 that there are 26 percent fewer nurses graduating from Vermont schools than six years ago. The report declared that Vermont is in the middle of a severe nursing shortage and must take serious and immediate steps to improve the situation.[9]

As the problem worsens, hospitals and other health care employers are finding new ways to retain and recruit nurses. Eighty-five percent of hospitals now pay a signing bonus to nurses (up from

67 percent in 1999).[10] Bonuses ranging from $2,000 to $15,000 have been reported at some hospitals, with the average being $6,500. Tuition reimbursement programs, child care subsidies, and even house-cleaning or lawn services are being used to attract nurses.[11]

All of the steps necessary to attract nurses are, of course, adding to the costs of operating a hospital. These increased costs will be added to hospital fees and then to premiums.

Nursing is hard work, and often done at inconvenient hours. It's easy to see why the profession is attracting fewer participants. Nurses want a working environment with reasonable staffing and workloads; collaborative relationships with physicians, managers, and other health professionals; and tools that will support their ability to deliver safe, quality patient care. We need nurses, so the solution will probably be at least partly economic: paying more money until the income levels offset many of the problems.

We Need More Therapists Too

The crisis in the supply of caregivers is not limited to nursing. For respiratory therapists, there are now 6,510 vacancies in acute care hospitals alone.[12] The number of jobs in respiratory therapy is projected to increase 42.6 percent by 2008, from 86,449 to 123,238.[13] It will take dollars to fix that situation—dollars that will also flow directly from premium increases.

The story is the same for X-ray technologists. The number enrolled in training programs declined by 26 percent from 1995 to 1999, and severe shortages are projected by 2010.[14] In fact, the government projects a shortage of 50,000 X-ray technologists by that year. There is a high level of irony in the fact that while there is miraculous new technology for diagnosing diseases, it might not be available to patients because of insufficient staff to run it.

As more people get cancer, they will very much want the possibility of cure by newer treatments. Many of those treatment programs will include radiation therapy. Will there be enough radiation therapists to perform these treatments? That's a serious concern. Graduated trainees in radiation therapy taking their certifying exams dropped by 58 percent from 1995 to 1999.

There will also be a major shortage of dentists. We currently graduate 4,000 new dentists each year, while 6,000 retire or die. This annual net loss of 2,000 dentists will create real problems not very far into the future.[15] This comes at a time when the demand will increase as a larger proportion of an aging population will keep their teeth and require dental work. The dental shortage will also result in the need for more dental hygienists because they will increasingly perform services now performed by dentists.

Nursing homes are also facing massive staff shortages. In some ways, nursing homes are the most troubled aspect of the entire U.S. care system. A combination of poor payment rates for Medicare and Medicaid patients, negative public perception of nursing homes, low wages and benefits, and a lack of training and advancement opportunities have produced a staffing crisis that will cause many nursing homes to shut over the next few years.[16] As our population ages, we will not have the care systems in place to deal with many older patients. Again, money could help fix that problem, but the government is the primary payer for the nursing home caregivers, and the government is both cheap and strapped for cash.

The demand for employees in many health care jobs will be strong in the next ten years, as indicated by the government projections of job growth from 1998 to 2008 by category of health care worker, shown in Figure 8.2. What impact will that have on health care costs?

One way of alleviating health care worker shortages will be to pay people more to take those jobs. We could fill our need in nursing jobs if we jumped the average salary. The average starting salary for a nurse in this country is about $39,000.[17] Other professionals with similar training can make significantly more money. Increasing nurse salaries could help by luring more people into the field.

Figure 8.2. Projected Job Growth in Selected Health Care Positions, 1998–2008

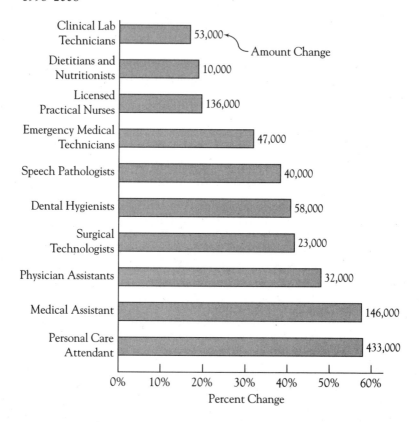

Source: U.S. Department of Health and Human Services, Health Resources and Services Administration, *Projected Supply, Demand, and Shortages of Registered Nurses: 2000–2020* (Washington, D.C.: U.S. Government Printing Office, July 2002).

Money isn't the only problem. Many health care jobs are hard work. The hours for care delivery are 24–7, not 9 to 5. You can't send all of the workers home from a hospital at 5:00 P.M. and let patients fend for themselves until morning. Someone has to work the night shifts. Someone has to work the swing shift. Those people all need to be paid.

Our nurses are also getting older. The average age of a working nurse is now forty-six.[18] Why is age relevant? If you have to help a 250-pound patient back into bed, would you rather do it when you are thirty years old or fifty?

Jobs Haven't Been Redesigned in a Decade

We also need to apply systems thinking much more effectively to health care. The job descriptions for many caregivers need to be rethought. Most job definitions for American caregivers were created decades ago. There is no other high-tech industry where the job descriptions today are the same for the key jobs as they were in 1980. Obviously, some serious work needs to be done to redesign some of the most critical jobs. Expecting an RN to do hands-on nursing while watching a dozen computer monitors and distributing complex regimens of medications to an ever-changing set of patients is not the best use of resources. We need to restructure the duties of various caregivers to maximize the benefit of each person's training and skill set.

Strategic use of technology—for example, automated medical records in hospitals—will help more than almost any other single tool or strategy. Currently, a lot of nurses' work load is involved in paper record keeping and in making sure all patients receive the right medicine, the right therapy, and the right care. That entire monitoring is manual. A well-designed computer system could help nurses do that job better and faster, allowing the nurses to focus more on patients in the process.

Restructuring will help, but it won't fix the problem. In each case, shortages will result in costs going up. The problem is less acute at the physician level, although there are shortages in some specialties. As we go forward, scarce specialties will command premium fees. Supply and demand will, as always, financially reward an undersupply.

All of those shortages are already pushing health care costs up. As we look forward, we can easily predict that caregiver wage levels will rise even further. Nurse unions, for example, are becoming increasingly assertive about both pay and work hour flexibility. That's an easy trend to understand. Health worker cost increases, like technology and drug cost increases, are not going away. The impact of those shortages on insurance premiums has already begun. It will accelerate over the next several years. Miracles cost money, and so do the staff necessary to make those miracles happen.

9

Medical Necessity Calls, Fee Cuts, and PR Errors—Not a Good Start

The vast majority of care delivered in the United States today is paid for by an HMO, a PPO, an insurance company using managed care techniques of one kind or another, or self-insured employers using some combination of HMO/PPO approaches and tactics. In about a decade, from 1990 to 2000, traditional fee-for-service insurance, with all patients able to seek care from any licensed provider, just about disappeared, replaced by various forms of managed care plans.

Six Unintended but Logical Reasons for Consumer Unhappiness

Usually when a product grows at an incredible rate and takes over a segment of the economy, that product basks in consumer popularity. Market success usually requires a direct linkage between consumer acceptance and volume growth. Health care, however, has followed a slightly different path. The fastest-growing product for health care financing in the past decade is also the product that has generated the most consumer unhappiness. Health plans, while generally popular with their own members, have come to have a fairly negative generic perception in the public mind.

How did that happen? A decade ago, health plans were celebrated by the public and media for improving benefits while cutting

117

costs. A decade later, the benefit expansions are all forgotten and the cost-containment techniques needed to achieve those expansions are resented, if not distrusted. So what happened in that decade to create that problem? We believe that question needs to be answered before the solutions for the next decade can be developed in ways that will achieve public acceptance.

Our answers might surprise you. We believe the answer to those questions relate primarily to six main issues:

- "Medical necessity" decisions

- Limited network choices

- Provider fee cut anger

- Experimental care exclusions

- Clumsy and overreaching HMO rules and processes

- Major misconceptions about HMO administrative costs and profits

Each of these issues needs to be understood and put in historical context before we can figure out what tools we have available as a society to solve today's health care cost crisis.

Medical Necessity Decisions

The first pressure point that creates stress and concern for significant numbers of people stems from the whole issue of "medical necessity." HMOs, almost without exception, use a standard called "medical necessity" to determine whether to cover specific benefits and payments for a given patient. Typically, all "medically necessary" treatments and procedures are paid for the patients by health plans. That creates goodwill. However, no payments are made for treatments and procedures that are not "medically necessary." The decisions that define medical necessity can create ill will and unhappiness. Medical necessity is a key concept that needs to be understood in order to appreciate how health plans are perceived by the public.

It is a hot issue. A significant number of people now object to health plans' making any medical necessity decisions. Medical necessity language is, however, in every HMO contract. How did that language get there? What is its purpose? What has been done to address the problems that arise from it?

Ironically, the original intent of the medical necessity standard was to expand benefits to improve patient care. The goal was to ensure that every patient received all medically necessary care.

The old pre-HMO indemnity insurance approach didn't cover medically necessary care. Those plans simply covered a limited list of predetermined procedures and usually placed a dollar limit on the fee to be paid for each procedure. The insurer set those fees. HMO coverage eliminated those fees as a benefit factor and substituted the concept of medical necessity. At the time, that was considered to be a consumer-friendly innovation and benefit expansion.

Here's the problem. To make that particular process work, someone has to determine what is and what is not medically necessary. Judgment calls are involved. The whole decision process is, unfortunately, often open to myriad levels of conflicts and misunderstandings. Most anti-HMO news stories focus on this particular issue, and most anti-HMO anecdotes deal with differences of opinion about the medical necessity definition. Both patients and doctors have had problems with some medical necessity decisions.

Limited Network Choices

The second reason for consumer unhappiness stems from the fact that network model HMOs typically offer care only from the doctors and hospitals that agree to accept the HMOs' fees. Some doctors reject those fees. That means that not every doctor in town is in every HMO. Consumers in some areas have ended up involuntarily changing doctors in order to receive full coverage from their employers.

Those forced changes have irritated many patients and further angered a large number of doctors.

Most HMOs have contracted care networks. A few plans work with a plan-exclusive set of providers. In either case, not all doctors in town are in the HMO, and some patients have to change physicians to be in the plan.

Provider Anger About Fee Cuts

The third point deals with absolutely understandable provider anger and unhappiness about discounted fees. That issue was discussed briefly in the chapter on provider consolidations and mergers. Angry providers talk publicly about quality of care, not about the quality of their personal paycheck. Ninety-nine out of a hundred provider-initiated private conversations between private, contracted providers of care and their health plans, however, focus exclusively on the issue of fees.

Experimental Care Exclusions

The fourth trigger point relates to the always touchy topic of experimental care. Neither the news media nor the public likes or accepts the standard exclusion in all insurance contracts for experimental care. Those cases generate a lot of publicity—all bad for the health plans.

Clumsy and Overreaching HMO Rules

The fifth cause for the widespread sense of generic guilt for HMOs comes from some unfortunate decisions made by some HMOs. Those decisions worked very directly to undermine consumer confidence in all HMO care. Some of those decisions, in retrospect, were ill advised. Some were clumsy. Some were stupid. A few were just plain bad. Those stories also need to be discussed and put into perspective. The current status of those issues also needs to be explained, because some of the more irritating problems that were part of the evolution of managed care in the 1990s have been dealt with and no longer exist in most settings.

Misconceptions of HMO Profits and Expenses

The sixth trigger point for consumer unhappiness is the overwhelming misconception on the part of consumers and news media about the size of HMO profits and HMO administrative expenses. When consumers believe that health plans achieve 20 to 30 percent profits by denying care and then use that money primarily to make plan executives filthy rich, it's hard to find many consumers who want health plans to expand their role in American health care. Less than 10 percent of the population currently guesses accurately when asked what health plan profits or operational costs actually are.

Separating Fiction from Facts

In total, the news media have used elements of all six factors as the foundation for continued anti-HMO stories. Those stories have been widely reported and have caused far too many people to believe the Hollywood scriptwriters all too easily when the writers insert HMO villains into their movies and TV shows. Until those issues are explained, discussed, and clearly understood, it will be almost impossible to design a health care solution for this country that has a reasonable chance of working.

Let's look at each of those issues starting with that nasty medical necessity issue. To do that, we need to take a historical perspective, going back to pre-HMO insurance coverage.

The Bad Old Days: Big Deductibles and Lifetime Benefits Caps

To understand the issue of medical necessity, it helps to have some historical perspective. Most people have been in some form of managed care plan or HMO for so long that they have forgotten what pre-HMO insurance coverage actually was like. People believe that in the days of traditional health insurance before HMOs existed, everything was fully covered. Not at all. Far from it.

The pre-HMO traditional insurance benefit packages were very different from HMO benefits, with old insurance plan benefits almost always much lower in scope. Typically, insurance companies had lists of approved procedures that they covered. Any procedures not on the lists were not covered. *Medical necessity* was a term invented to free caregivers from that rigid list. All care that an HMO patient needed, provided it was medically necessary, was to be covered.

The old indemnity insurance plans were restrictive in a number of ways. There was a time, for example, and only a few years ago, when the standard pre-HMO health insurance contract contained an important cost limiting benefit restriction provision called the *lifetime maximum*. It meant just what the name implies. If you, as a patient, needed more care than the lifetime maximum allowed for in your contract, then your insurance coverage simply ran out. Past that point, you were on your own. Financially naked.

Typically, those lifetime maximums in traditional pre-HMO insurance contracts ranged from $50,000 to $100,000 per person per lifetime. If you were sick enough to spend more than $100,000 on care, that was too bad. All care costs after that point were your personal responsibility. Lifetime maximums helped reduce the cost of insurance coverage.

In that same pre-HMO era, health insurance coverage paid only fixed fees for each procedure. If your doctor or hospital charged more than the preset insurance fee for a procedure or service, the additional cost was also entirely your responsibility. You paid it in cash.

In the 1980s, most pre-HMO health insurance plans also included front-end deductibles. Five hundred dollar deductibles were the norm for most medium-sized and small employer groups. (Some insurance companies set deductibles at $1,000 per person.) After you paid the full deductible yourself, you usually also personally paid 20 percent of any remaining bill (plus any fee overages). Some deductibles were annual. Some actually were per admission, so you could pay several deductibles each year. If your deductible was $500, in other words, you would pay your own out-of-pocket money for the first $500 worth of care. Then your insurer would start paying part of the bill using a fee schedule set by them. You would then also share in the remaining cost, paying a copayment equal to 20 percent of the fee schedule (plus any additional costs if your doctor's fee schedule was higher than your insurance companies' fee schedule).

Then, if you were really sick, your coverage would literally run out. It would end entirely at $50,000 or $100,000, or at whatever lifetime maximum level you or your employer had purchased.

Some plans, which were considered very generous, ran the lifetime maximum payment level up to $250,000 or even $500,000. A few even offered—for additional premium—a million dollar cap. In each case, however, when personal care costs hit the cap, the patient was on his or her own. That was the standard model of pre-HMO insurance care in the 1980s.

HMOs' Far Richer Benefits

Then HMOs came along with a very different approach. HMOs guaranteed care, not just specific fee payments for a predetermined schedule of procedures. Lifetime maximums disappeared. HMOs offered, in effect, unlimited benefits for all medically necessary care, including prevention services and physical exams that had not been covered by most traditional insurance companies. It was a revolutionary change, and people loved it. Patients traded very limited benefits for unlimited benefits. Lifetime maximums disappeared. Fee schedules disappeared. Deductibles also disappeared. HMOs paid full benefits from the start.

Copayments almost disappeared. Some HMOs did use small copayments generally as per visit charges. Usually, however, these copays were less than ten dollars. In early years, they typically ran five dollars or less. Many were initially under a dollar. (Fifty cent prescription drug copayments, for example, were not uncommon in 1990–1991.)

In other words, the new HMO benefit packages were unquestionably richer and more complete than the traditional insurance plans they replaced. When actuaries calculated the benefit difference, the mathematically weighted value of typical HMO benefits was about 27 percent higher than the typical pre-HMO insurer benefit package. But HMOs cost less, and often a lot less. How could more benefits cost less?

More Benefits for Fewer Dollars

As discussed previously, HMOs used their patient volume to negotiate fees with providers of care. These fees usually resulted in deep discounts for the HMOs that helped offset the cost of the richer HMO benefits. They offered more care for less money in effect. Over half of the HMO premium savings came from these discounts.

The other half of the savings that allowed HMOs to open up benefits fully and eliminate those burdensome copays, deductibles, fee schedules, and lifetime maximums resulted from the HMOs' ability to provide benefits only for medically necessary care. "Medically necessary" meant they would pay for whatever care was actually needed, but they would not pay for unnecessary care.

This new medical necessity concept had a huge initial impact on costs because quite a bit of medical care in the era before HMOs was incredibly wasteful and inefficient. Pre-HMO doctors would, for example, routinely admit patients to hospitals for overnight stays simply to take X rays. Those totally unnecessary hospital admissions added hundreds, sometimes thousands, of dollars to each patient's bill but added absolutely no value in care. It made a lot more sense to have most of those X rays done in a much less expensive (and generally much more convenient) outpatient setting.

The new network model HMOs required doctors to perform these X rays in nonhospital settings. "Medical necessity," not "medical convenience," was the rule used to determine the site of care.

The X ray itself was medically necessary, so it was paid for in full by the HMO. The X-ray-based hospital stay, however, had absolutely no medical necessity, so the in-hospital stay was not covered.

Overall hospital use was cut in half by HMOs. Millions of dollars were saved. Patients avoided being injured or infected in hospitals. Costs went down, and care got better. Everybody won, except the hospitals, which lost a lot of easy revenue.

The starting list of wasteful and medically unnecessary processes was huge. Pre-HMO doctors had been routinely admitting patients to hospitals on Friday nights for tests to be conducted on Monday. That added two or three totally unnecessary hospital days to the hospital bill for no added care value. Maternity stays used to run a week or more for a normal delivery. HMOs reduced the length of stay for maternity to three days and then to two. The very best medical experts said that any inpatient days beyond two for a normal birth were not only medically unnecessary but were at least slightly dangerous to mother and child. (Recent hospital safety studies have verified that fear, as everyone now knows.)

Overall, hospital use was cut in half by HMOs' simply saying, "We won't pay for any hospital stays that serve no medical purpose." That saved a lot of money.

So partly as a result of applying medical necessity standards to care and partly due to HMO-negotiated discounts in provider fees, the scope of coverage and benefits increased significantly under HMOs while the costs to members and patients decreased.

Again, that can be seen as a win for the patients. But it was a real problem for many doctors whose fees were cut and for hospitals whose patient volume was reduced.

Any Judgment Is Open to Challenge

Almost without exception, the patient came out well ahead in the deal. Premiums for a much more robust set of benefits were cheaper than the premiums for the old $500 deductible, 80 percent/20 percent insurance plans. But, interestingly, although the new medical necessity rule was a success in many ways, it also ended up creating a whole new series of issues and some big problems for HMO patients. Even when the patient came out way ahead on benefits, the process of adjudicating what was medically necessary sometimes created complications and tension between members and claims processors.

In retrospect, it's easy to see why. Take the issue of wheelchair coverage as a typical example. Apply a standard of medical necessity to wheelchair coverage. A traditional pre-HMO insurance plan would pay only a flat fee for a wheelchair—typically $500 or, in better policies, $1,000. A patient needing a wheelchair would find the chair, pay for it, and then send a claim to the insurer. Let's say that the patient had the best available pre-HMO coverage: a $1,000 chair allowance. If the wheelchair that the patient selected cost $1,000 or less, the traditional insurer paid the full cost (less, of course, any copays or deductibles that the patient had yet to pay). If the new wheelchair cost $4,000, the pre-HMO insurer still paid only $1,000. The patient paid the remaining $3,000. The arithmetic was simple. No judgments were involved. The payment level was rigid, clearly defined, and fixed.

That old pre-HMO benefit arrangement was easy to calculate, easy for everyone to understand, and easy to pay. It was also pretty limited. If the patient needed a special chair with many features and the cost of the chair hit $10,000, then the patient was out of luck. The insurer still paid only $1,000, and the patient had to pay the rest out of pocket. Patients didn't fight with the insurance company on this point, however, because the limitation was totally clear. The whole process was easy for all parties to understand. It did not involve any decisions by anyone other than the patient and the doctor about which wheelchair to buy.

The new HMO wheelchair benefits, by contrast, were much richer. They covered all costs for the medically necessary "service" (the chair) instead of paying a fixed fee. So for any given patient, medical necessity, not a rigid and limited fee schedule, determined the HMO benefit level. If the patient needed a $10,000 chair, the HMO paid all $10,000.

The New Process Required a Decision

Of course, someone at the HMO had to decide what level of wheelchair was medically necessary. That isn't anywhere near as simple as just paying a limited flat fee.

And this is where the problems started. Each health plan set its own rules, guidelines, and standards to make those decisions. How crippled must someone be to get a motorized wheelchair? How incapacitated must a person be to have a head brace built in to the chair? At what point should the wheelchair have a radio built in? A phone? Sculpted cushions? Snow tires?

In quite a few cases, the patient wanted a deluxe chair of some kind, but the plan said, "According to our assessment of your health condition, you are medically entitled to a basic chair. So that's what we will get for you, a basic chair, a $1,500 basic chair."

Making these decisions is obviously a miserable, thankless process. Disagreements about definitions abound. Even with guidelines in place, the best-intentioned people can differ on those judgment calls, and they often did. As time went on, those disagreements increasingly came into public view. Some patients have gone to court. Some have gone to various legislators, pointing out that they personally believed they needed a fully motorized chair and the miserly plan would pay only for a lousy basic chair instead. The plan, of course, generally sounds like an unfeeling villain when the testimony is coming from a person in the wheelchair.

Anytime the person testifying against you is in a wheelchair, you know you're in trouble.

So, ironically, although the new benefit approach actually provided better and much more flexible wheelchair coverage for just about all patients, the mere opportunity to differ about chair selection has created real morale, trust, and satisfaction problems for both the patients and the plans.

For most of those kinds of situations, the plans could have saved themselves a lot of grief by simply saying, "We're going back to using the old insurance model, maybe with slightly better benefits. You pick the chair. We'll pay $2,000 for whatever chair you pick. That's the full benefit. Use it well."

That approach to many HMO benefits would have avoided untold thousands of hassles, ducked a deluge of debates, and eliminated most of the tension relative to wheelchair and other durable medical equipment choices. It would have simply removed the potential for conflict. It would also have simplified administration, because the entire wheelchair benefit adjudication process would have simply been to say yes or no rather than "which chair." "Which" takes a lot more staff time than either yes or no.

"Parental" Medical Directors Designed "Medical Necessity" Benefits

The plans, however, stuck by their commitment to the medically necessary standard. This is, in part, because the first HMO-like health plans were started by people who were passionately committed to improving and expanding benefits. The first plans believed so strongly in providing the full medically necessary benefit set that the new approach was almost always locked into all member contracts for the full range of HMO benefits. It was even, in some states, locked into law. The first plans strongly supported those laws and helped get them passed.

Why did those first HMOs insist on medical necessity as the guideline for all benefits? The answer is, in part, ideology and, in part, innocence.

One reason for the naiveté of the early HMO contract writers on that particular point was that almost all of the early health plans were consumer focused and even consumer owned. They were created by health care reformers. Most of these plans were nonprofit and were, in effect, consumer coalitions for better health. In the case of Kaiser Permanente, these decisions were made entirely by physicians who were members of the Permanente Medical Group. In the case of the member-governed health plans (like Group Health), the plans hired medical directors who also personally believed that they, as plan physicians, were true and pure consumer advocates. Those medical directors and Kaiser Permanente physicians believed they each worked directly for the members and that they were uniquely qualified to make competent and highly ethical medical necessity decisions on benefits for consumers. These doctors also believed consumers would gratefully and willingly accept the doctor's status as an objective decision maker.

Medical necessity may be purely intentioned. It may actually be a wonderful, consumer-friendly approach. But it has inherent and obvious built-in conflicts that cannot be avoided for even the best-intentioned, purest-hearted health plan. It's human nature that some people will always want a bigger wheelchair. Any system that offers an open checkbook and then inserts an invisible and remote decision maker, who regulates access to that checkbook, has a big potential problem built right in.

That conflict always existed to some degree. It was less of a problem in the early days of health plans when it was very clear to members that the plans were nonprofit and offering very complete benefits. It is more heated today when most HMOs are now for profit. Consumers sometimes wonder what impact the need for profit has on individual medical necessity decisions. Being for profit does not mean that plans make bad decisions on these issues, but it does mean that both consumers and the media are more likely to wonder about the objectivity of the people making those various decisions.

What's Behind the Dissatisfaction

These six key issues have had a seismic impact on perceptions of "managed care." Understanding the context in which these six key issues evolved can point the way to potential solutions.

The Future of Medical Necessity Must Be Decided

What can plans, nonprofit and for-profit alike, do about this issue? Should they simply abandon any standard and just pay for any wheelchair that any patient might want? That would resolve the plan objectivity issue. It would, however, not help the cost of premium issue. Costs would explode. And so would premiums.

If every wheelchair patient gets the deluxe $10,000 model, then those costs will drive even higher premiums. As an alternative, plans could go in exactly the opposite direction: end the tension and avoid the subjectivity stress by simply returning to the old pre-HMO world of defined and limited preset cash payments for a specific list of health care goods and services. That approach could cost less than a medical necessity approach and would eliminate all of those troublesome judgment calls.

The ultimate answer will probably involve a combination of defined services and specific limited benefits. That's really the only way for the plans to avoid the ongoing animosity and stress. Plans cannot afford to have members angry, but plans also cannot afford to provide unlimited medically unnecessary care.

That's the medical necessity dilemma: the only way to offer unlimited benefits for an affordable price is to have some form of rigorously applied medical necessity clause for most elements of care. The system cannot afford a return to five-day maternity stays or inpatient CAT scans for sore shoulders. But consumers are increasingly unwilling to have plans make those medical necessity decisions. The only affordable and practical alternative to medical necessity may well be to bring back significant benefit limitations and use very clear benefit definitions in the contracts. Clarity must replace subjectivity whenever possible.

In any case, a decade or more of medical necessity decisions has already caused enough consumers sufficient concern to be a major factor in the current debate about HMOs.

Limited Network Choices: Why Isn't the Doctor I Want in My Plan?

Another factor that arouses consumer ire in many markets is that HMOs tell patients which doctors they may use for care. That is, they impose network limitations.

Interestingly, consumers were less upset by this in the early days of HMOs. When HMOs were first offered, they were always offered side by side with traditional insurance plans. Although these traditional plans usually cost a lot more money, patients still had a choice. They could choose the smaller HMO network and save money, or they could choose the larger insurance network, pick all of their own doctors, and pay more for their premium. People who selected HMOs in that era did so willingly, and they almost always accepted the inevitable trade-off of a smaller network as part of their personal purchasing criteria.

In some areas of the country, that practice of offering multiple plans to employees still exists. In other areas, employers are reducing the number of plans offered or offering only a single plan to their employees. That single plan seldom, if ever, has all local providers in their network.

So why do health plans have limited networks? In some of the traditional staff and group model plans, the networks are an integral and exclusive part of the health plan operation. In other plans, the networks are composed of nonexclusive providers—limited to those providers who agree, under contract, to accept the HMO's payment levels for care. Those payment levels are typically a good bit lower than the "retail" prices charged by those same providers.

In order to negotiate the best possible fees, the HMOs generally had to play providers off one another. Only those physicians and hospitals that accepted the HMO fee discounts actually ended up in any given HMO provider network.

Those restricted care networks were the real beginning of the anti-HMO backlash in the minds of many consumers. As noted, it also started the full emotional anti-HMO backlash from the perspective of many doctors. Contracted and deeply discounted doctors quite often shared their unhappiness with their patients.

So that was the second reason for the growing sense on the part of many people that health plans were somehow "generically guilty." Unhappy physicians told their patients to be distrustful of HMOs.

Provider Anger About Fee Cuts

The third major cause of consumer unhappiness with HMOs springs, we believe, from doctor-patient conversations. As we noted earlier, many physicians grew to be unhappy with health plans for two primary reasons. The doctors who signed these steeply discounted HMO contracts were often deeply unhappy because they were now being paid less money for each unit of care. Many of those doctors felt impoverished by the process. (Some defined impoverishment at a fairly lofty level, but others did see real and painful cuts in their take-home pay.)

Doctors who didn't sign HMO contracts were also very angry because they lost some of their patients to the HMOs. New HMO enrollees who used to go to those doctors for care could no longer do so. Instead, they had to choose a doctor affiliated with the plan. Quite a few doctors, then, for obvious reasons, began to speak disparagingly about HMOs to the patients. Since most physicians didn't want to complain to patients about making less money, many decided to complain instead about HMO impact on care, whether or not any quality issues existed. Much of the public's negative perception about HMOs resulted in part from those conversations.

The quality issues raised in those conversations tended to be nonspecific but heartfelt. One can make a fairly strong argument that health plan actions have improved both care access and care quality for a large number of patients, but in the mid-1990s, no one made that argument.

As near as we can tell, none of the exam room conversations between doctors and patients ever focused on discounted fees.

Experimental Care Exclusions Were Covered

The fourth reason for HMOs' being judged generically guilty, experimental care exclusions, has already been covered in sufficient detail in Chapter Three. People want HMOs to cover experimental care. No HMO or insurer now provides benefits for unproven care.

We raise this issue again in this chapter because those issues do tend to create major concern with some regularity. The number of actual experimental care cases is, in total, quite small. But when the patients involved are very sick or dying and are put in the media limelight, these cases take on a visibility far out of proportion to their actual numbers. Public opinion is clearly shaped; plans are perceived as denying hope to dying people.

In truth, plans spend huge amounts of money—literally billions of dollars—saving people's lives. Heroic care is common and covered, but those stories seldom get told, pushed out by anecdotes about denied coverage for experimental care cases. Those stories do not help reassure people about the care they will receive from their HMO when they need it.

This isn't speculation. Research shows that people watching the TV stories miss the point in each that the denied care is experimental. Most viewers believe that the care is rejected by the plan because it is expensive. Large numbers of people now believe that plans deny any care that costs a lot of money. In the real world, that isn't true. There are no plan exclusions for expensive care, just exclusions for experimental care. Expensive care happens all the time, and even extremely expensive care that is enough to run premiums up to nearly $1,000 a month in family coverage. But those cases are seldom, if ever, publicized.

Again, as with medical necessity definitions and wheelchairs, plans cannot win this argument. It may make more sense for them to take a whole new approach, selling optional coverage for experimental care to anyone who wants to spend the additional money to buy it. Then, if experimental care is denied, the plan could say, "We offered Mr. Smith coverage for experimental care. He chose to save $30 a month and decided not to buy it. He therefore doesn't have it." It would be fascinating to see how the news media would respond to that answer.

For now, however, experimental care is not covered, and the news stories about those relatively rare cases have a major negative impact on the public perception of HMOs.

Clumsy and Overreaching HMO Rules

Some of the criticism directed against health plans is based on mis-understandings. Some is based on inaccurate descriptions of plan behavior. And some is deserved, based on plans "going one bridge too far" in some areas of care. When that has happened, people have noticed. Public responses to overreaching HMO rules have been negative and long lasting. To understand how and why some plans reached over the bridge, we need to remember the evolu-tionary process for medical necessity decision making.

Traditional insurance companies never questioned the validity of any care. If a licensed provider did it and the procedure was one that was specifically listed on the insurer's fee schedule, the claim was paid.

HMOs took a different road. They began to administer the med-ical necessity provisions built into both the provider and patient contracts. In the process, plans began to manage care.

The first managed care efforts were fairly simple, easy to do, ex-tremely useful, and painfully obvious. HMOs, for example, asked their doctors to stop admitting otherwise healthy patients to hos-pitals twenty-four to forty-eight hours before surgery. Those patients had no medical reason to be in the hospital. In most cases, they were there for the doctors' convenience.

The cost problem was that hospitals tended to charge for a full day of care for those patients, even though the patients received no real care. That approach was profitable for hospitals but extremely expensive for insurers. It increased and inflated premium rates. Elim-inating that totally unnecessary hospital day saved the new health plans many millions of dollars and reduced the premiums charged to health plan members.

Doctors and hospitals didn't protest those initial types of "man-aged care" decisions because the HMOs were so obviously right. Money was being wasted. Anyone who looked could see it.

That was just the beginning. Waste was everywhere. HMOs eliminated the chest X ray that every hospital patient used to receive upon admission. That X ray had supposedly once helped hospital officials discover undiagnosed tuberculosis, but it had long since become merely a profitable billing opportunity for most hospitals.

HMOs began looking at hospital lengths of stay. There were initially some very easy targets in that area. No one could give a medical reason for mothers' spending a full week in the hospital after the normal birth of a healthy baby, for example. So health plans reduced the length of stay to four days, then three days, then two days. Nothing medical was being done for the mothers in those extra three or four days. Many mothers loved the hospital days, however, particularly if their home environment was hectic or not supportive. A week in the hospital could sometimes be a welcome respite, particularly when there was no real medical reason for being there. Nevertheless, a reduction to two days was accepted, though with some grumbling.

The first level of hospital stay reductions were win-win situations for the plans and the patients. Eventually, however, all the clear and easy reductions had been made. Looking for another round of savings, the plans started to fine-tune the process. That's when the trouble started. Many plans, for example, attempted to reduce the maternity stay to one day in the hospital.

Those plans had good medical science on their side, but a very bad sense of public relations or patient satisfaction.

The One-Day OB Stay Was a Major Error

The situation immediately crossed the line from stressful to unacceptable. Again, top medical minds said a one-day maternity stay was fine, even preferable, assuming there had been no complications in the birth and there was appropriate home care follow-up. Recent studies have confirmed that assessment. Public opinion, however, said that a one-day stay was a crime, an evil plot created by greedy and unfeeling HMOs to save money at the expense of a new mother and her tiny, helpless child.

In retrospect, anyone in the HMO world who thought that a one-day OB stay was a public relations battle that could have been won was a fool. There were quite a number in the industry who held the somewhat arrogant and close-minded belief that pure medical science was the only standard that should be used to make those sorts of hospital use decisions. The public perception—very reasonably—is that labor is an exhausting process. Sending mothers home to care for a newborn after a day's stay was an unpopular decision. Issues came into play that were not purely medical.

We were wrong. Maintaining patient trust is a key part of the healing and therapeutic process. Trust is far too valuable to be ignored in favor of pure science. That maternity decision and a couple others like it damaged both patient and community trust. Once impaired, trust is pretty hard to regain.

That was one of the HMO industry's darkest hours. HMO medical leaders were, in fact, listening to the experts who believed that a second day of maternity stay was unnecessary and a waste of members' premiums for normal deliveries. The plans at that time somewhat insensitively believed that medical science should and would trump public opinion on all such issues and that reason would soon prevail.

It was a bad call. That's not the way any marketplace works or the way people think. We forgot that customers' opinions are an important part of any business decision, particularly in a service industry.

The public backlash was immense. Politicians seized on the issue and galloped forward to protect mothers. The media loved doing those stories featuring moms who were forced out of the hospitals' warm arms before the sun had set on the day after their delivery. Plans suffered a black eye that has never quite healed, a deterioration of public trust that has yet to be rebuilt.

At that point, a spontaneous medical counterattack on several other hospital use issues began. The tinder was ready, waiting for a spark. For example, community doctors originally offered no public objection to plan decisions such as reducing the length of stay for gallbladder surgery from two weeks to one week. Everyone knew two weeks was excessive, wasteful, and even dangerous. But when plans tried to turn the seven-day gallbladder stay into a five-day stay, medical judgment issues came into play. Reasonable and caring and highly skilled doctors could argue either side of the point. Gray areas were reached. Plans do not and will not win debates when areas are gray and the other party to the debate is the patient's own physician. No one argued for a return to the gross wastefulness of the 1980s, but new lines were drawn about exactly how much waste could and should be removed from today's system.

How Many Gag Clauses Were There?

With issues like one-day maternity stays fanning the flames, the media began to do a series of anti–health plan stories in the late 1990s.

The accuracy level of those news reports was not particularly consistent. Perhaps the most frustrating and damaging media misrepresentation in the mid-1990s concerned purported "physician gag clauses." An East Coast physician held a widely publicized press conference to announce that his HMO had asked him to sign a frightening contractual clause that would have prevented him from having discussions with patients about any care options not approved by his HMO. He was outraged. So were the news media. Very shortly thereafter, so was the American public. National news magazines ran cover stories asking, "What Doesn't Your HMO Doctor Tell You?" Patient paranoia levels soared across the country. Public anger exploded. The U.S. government investigated to see how widespread the problem was.

A careful investigation by the U.S. government proved that the gag clause problem did not exist. Extraordinarily few health plans ever had an unfortunate and overreaching gag clause like the misguided plan mentioned earlier. Gag clauses, in reality, were a myth.

The media, sadly, almost totally ignored a subsequent government investigatory report showing that no other gag clauses existed anywhere. No one wrote a story staying, "HMOs do not gag your doctor. Your doctor can tell you everything." Dozens of states actually passed strongly worded antigag clause legislation, often at the request of local HMOs and HMO associations that all actively opposed any possible use of those clauses.[1] All plans wanted to be very clear in their absolute opposition to anyone acting in that manner.

Unfortunately, the media reported on the number of legislatures that passed such laws, with most stories implying that widespread HMO practices made the laws necessary. None of the media stories noted that the issue had been proved to be a myth or that, in most states, local HMOs were the organizations pushing the legislation.[2]

Over the past several years, script writers for TV shows and movies have managed to create stories in which HMOs played the role of villains. In one movie, an HMO was vilified for forcing a child to get all of his asthma care from an emergency room. No HMO in America would ever use an emergency room as the routine site for a child's asthma care. The facts, however, were not the issue. A generic sense of mistrust was the issue. The scripts reflected that mistrust.

Americans Want Their Own Doctor's Judgment to Prevail

A definite learning process has gone on in the HMO industry. At one point, for some types of care, some HMOs probably did make people unhappy by imposing the judgment of their medical leaders over the judgment of the patients' own doctors. The plans would argue that at worst, those were areas where both opinions were equally medically valid. That "equal validity" isn't an argument that sells with the public.

In our personal plans, that never happened. The Kaiser Permanente physicians have always set their own care standards. So has the HealthPartners Medical Group. But there were other instances where certain judgments were made that could lead to the kind of concerns that resulted in those movie scripts.

Americans gladly accept the elimination of medical waste. Americans accept and even embrace programs to improve care systematically. They do not, however, accept a doctor other than the one they have chosen making their medical decisions in areas where the issue isn't pure science but rather informed medical opinion and relative expertise.

That is exactly as it should be. That's the optimal way of looking at the doctor-patient relationship. That isn't to say that the plans shouldn't act on behalf of the members to improve care, particularly in settings where the plans offer the only systematic quality improvement. In many cases, plans have made a real difference in care quality. Getting rid of bad drugs improved care. Eliminating unnecessary C-sections improved care. Plan physicians can tell dozens of similar stories.

The problem came in figuring out when the issues had crossed the line from obvious waste to optimal judgment.

In any case, experience was necessary for managed care to start to figure out where waste reduction ended and interference with care began. Mistakes were sometimes made. The learning curve for some plans was fairly steep. The process took a few years to evolve, but that evolution has occurred. At this point, the plans are much more sophisticated on each of these points and have moved to a new level of review.

The best plans now strongly encourage the use of guidelines that help define best care rather than using rules intended to achieve lowest-cost care. The jury is still out on whether the guidelines will, in the end, cost more or less than the rules. But care will probably be better with guidelines, and the whole system can function as a team rather than as dueling subcomponents.

Misconceptions About HMO Profits and Administrative Costs

The sixth reason for consumer distrust of HMOs is a major public misperception about the percentage of the premium dollar that goes for HMO profits, HMO administrative expenses, and HMO executive salaries. Surveys in Minnesota have indicated that most consumers believe that HMO profits range from 10 to 30 percent of premium and that HMO administrative costs range as high as 40 percent of premium. National surveys have come up with similar results. If those numbers were true, they would be a major reason to shut down HMOs as quickly as possible. Such numbers would almost be a criminal misuse of the health care dollar.

In fact, HMO profits range from losses of a few percent to gains of up to 5 or 6 percent. Profits higher than that are extremely rare. It's interesting to note that a profit of 5 percent is one-sixth of the public belief.

HMO administrative costs range from 3 to 20 percent of premium, with the average number closer to 12 percent. That's roughly one-fourth of the most common public perception.

So why, if administrative costs are actually relatively low and plan profits are even lower, does the public believe that these sums are criminally high? Again, the news media can take some of the credit. When plan profits rose from a national average of 1 percent to a national average of 3 percent, the headlines didn't say, "Plan Profits Climb Slightly." Three percent is, in fact, a minuscule profit level in many industries. Journalists could have pointed that out. Most newspapers run at a 10 percent to 30 percent profit level or they go out of business.

Reporters didn't mention that fact or make that comparison. Instead, the headlines shouted "HMO Profits Climb 200 Percent." Two hundred percent sounds like a really big number, an unconscionably big number, even an alarming number. But when the smoke clears, that alarmingly big number is actually just a 3 percent profit this year compared to a 1 percent profit last year.

Whether or not the 3 percent profit makes sense, it's pretty clear that a 3 percent profit is not causing today's 20 percent annualized increases in health care costs. Do the math. It isn't complicated.

HMO Administrative Costs Are Below
Traditional Insurance Costs

It is particularly frustrating to some HMO executives to hear plans attacked for administrative cost when HMOs actually take a smaller percentage of administrative dollars from their premium than did the traditional insurance companies who preceded HMOs.

For individuals and small groups, traditional non-HMO insurers have usually charged from 20 to 40 percent of premiums for administration, numbers that are, ironically, as bad as the public mistakenly believes HMO administrative costs to be. A return to the "good old days" of traditional insurance actually would mean a return to huge administrative costs and waste.

Plans Have Learned over Time

Plans have been burned by all of those issues relative to public credibility. Experimental care, medical necessity, and closed networks have all generated bad public relations and lower trust levels.

Plans have learned from that whole process. Different plans are responding differently. Some have cut way back on the levels of screening they do relative to hospital use. Others have evolved from rules to guidelines, influencing better care rather than dictating it. Those actions will all help restore plan credibility over time, but not very quickly. The legacy of the one-day maternity stay will not fade for quite a while, and some portions of the public will never forget it. Those people will continue to find all plans generically guilty.

HMOs Will Prosper but Won't Be Loved

What does the current public attitude toward HMOs mean for the costs of health care in this country? It means that the general public will not automatically turn to HMOs to solve the new explosion in health care costs.

Buyers, however, don't have any viable alternatives. They don't have any other effective tool to use if they want to keep providing benefits to their employees. Employers and the government see some version of health plans as an important player in the upcoming health care cost battle.

As an industry, the more innovative and competent HMOs will probably do well over the next three to five years because the cost pressures in today's health care economy will force buyers to use every available mechanism. As outlined in Chapter Eight, only HMOs can provide most of those tools.

Those of us who know what incredible success can be achieved with the HMO tool kit will continue to promote systematic best care, outcomes measurement, patient-focused chronic care, and increased individual patient involvement in care decisions. We don't expect any of this to be reported in the public media for a few years, but that won't keep the plans from using those tools to improve the quality and value of care. The truth, we believe, will eventually be told.

For Now, Relaxing Rigor Is the Rule

For now, most health plans are responding to public unhappiness by reducing their cost controls. There is a definite loosening of focus on lengths of hospital stays, appropriate site of procedures, drug formularies, and all of the other tools that helped keep costs under control but caused consumers some unhappiness. Relaxed plan rigor is allowing the return of some unnecessary costs to the system, costs that are already being charged to consumers in premiums.

Some plans will reduce specific benefits significantly to offset the disappearance of medical necessity as a tool. The old fixed payment insurance benefit set will return for a great many Americans because those benefit limitations offer premium savings.

Americans want full benefits and no restrictions. That won't happen. There's no such thing as a free lunch.

What are our choices for the future?

10

So Why Don't We Just Go to
a Single-Payer System and
Save Bucks Like the Brits?

As we said in the Introduction to this book, if current trends
continue, America will find itself facing a series of health care
crises within two years. Most employers will not be able to continue
subsidizing the care expenses of their employees. Shifting the cost
to employees will create anger and fear—anger directed against
whoever created this mess and fear of being unable to afford care in
the future.

A great many smaller employers will drop coverage altogether,
causing the number of uninsured Americans to skyrocket. It's not
impossible to envision a scenario that adds another 10 to 20 million Americans to the ranks of the uninsured within those years.
All in all, that's a climate that will lead to people wanting things to
change.

So what alternatives do we have? One option would be to follow the trend of every other industrialized nation and create a
government-run single-payer health system. A few years ago, that
option was unthinkable for health planners in this country. There
is, however, evidence that sizable percentages of Americans are now
ready to consider having this country move to a single-payer form
of government-run health insurance.

It's easy to see why that might seem like a good idea. Other countries spend a lot less money on health care than the United States
does, and most end up creating universal coverage for all citizens in

the process. The two systems that most American single-payer advocates mention most are the British and Canadian systems. Both offer full coverage for all citizens at a cost significantly lower than the U.S. health care expenditure level.

In practical terms, it might be easier for the United States to emulate the Canadian model. The British system requires direct government ownership of very large portions of the care system. We would need to have the government directly own 80 percent of the hospitals and employ more than 80 percent of all U.S. physicians, for example, to copy the British approach. The process necessary to transfer ownership of the private health care economy into government property and government employees would be massive, and the up-front expense of having the government buy that entire infrastructure would be prohibitive. It's hard to imagine a return-on-investment scenario where the government could pay a fair price to take over the private care system and then achieve enough subsequent savings to make the massive investment worthwhile.

It's even harder to imagine a scenario where the government could take over the entire care system and then somehow manage it very well. The government has great strengths, but actual operational management isn't always one of them.

The Canadian system, in contrast to the British approach, allows for slightly more private ownership and, like our typical American insurance model, makes most payments to medical providers through a per incident fee schedule rather than through salaries. Hospitals are government owned in Canada. Most physician practices are not.

Either approach has the very real potential to save money, but—and this is the key issue—we need to be honest with ourselves. We will save money with a single-payer system here only if we use the exact same techniques those other countries use to save money for health care. They don't use magic to hold costs in line. They use government budgets. Real budgets. Rationing budgets. They each ration care. In each of those countries, care runs out when the budget runs out. More than 50,000 people are currently waiting more than a year for hospital admissions in Great Britain. Hospitals in Canada frequently stop admitting nonemergency patients in December, when their funds run out.

That type of hard-nosed decision about limiting the availability of care may be an insurmountable political challenge in this country. It's not clear right now that Americans are ready to have their personal health care budgeted or rationed by anyone.

The world pattern is pretty clear. In any country where the government is responsible for the cost of care, the government limits the availability of that care to the amount of money available in a year's government budget. This isn't a theoretical point. A single-payer system would put our government in the same position.

Our Government Already Rations Care

Some American advocates of a single-payer system claim that our government would not use those techniques and approaches. "Our government would not ration care," they say. "We'd continue to have all of the wonderful care we have today, just with a lower cost. Rationing wouldn't be an American single-payer approach. We'd use a different approach to saving money."

Is that true? Would our government uniquely choose not to ration care if given a choice?

Unfortunately, we already have the answer to that question. Just look at drug coverage for Medicare patients. If you doubt for a moment that our government would also decide to ration care if and when that care becomes a government expense, just look at the issue of prescription drugs and Medicare. Seniors need their drugs more than any other segment of our population. Why don't they have coverage of drugs by Medicare? Government rationing, pure and simple. Our government doesn't want the expense, so it rations drugs, just like every other government that takes on the responsibility of paying for care. Medicaid is another area where our government has been tested relative to its ability to rise above rationing as a response to health care cost pressure. State after state is cutting benefits, cutting coverage, and reducing eligibility. The people being deprived of care are our poorest, neediest citizens.

So the answer is already clear.

Will our government ration care to balance our total care budgets if the government somehow becomes the single payer for all care? Yes. Obviously. Our government has already failed the rationing test, and badly.

Are Americans ready to have the government ration our personal care to cut the costs of care? Probably not yet. But times change. When premiums cut badly into the take-home pay of American citizens and the number of uninsured grows, that balance could shift, and a government-run system might start looking more attractive. That new coverage would not be free, of course. An American single-payer system would need to have a tax-based payment source.

At this point, with a faltering economy, it's not at all clear that American citizens are ready to bear the new taxes that would be required so that the government would have enough money to pay for all of the care now available in this country. It would take significant new taxes simply to sustain our current care delivery system at today's levels. That new tax burden would be significant. But it would be necessary because a single-payer, government-run program for universal health care would require the U.S. government to come up with enough tax money to pay for everyone's care.

How much money would the government need?

The annual tax burden in Great Britain right now for health care is roughly $1,763 per capita.[1] (Note that this figure assumes that all health spending in the U.K. is "public." According to the Organization for Economic Cooperation and Development, 81 percent of U.K. total health expenditures are "public," which reduces the 2000 U.K. heath-related tax burden to $1,428.) That tax burden wouldn't come close to covering the U.S. health care expenses for an American single-payer system.

Here's why. The current annual cost of the U.S. health care system, private and public, is $1.4 trillion.[2] Divide this number by the total number of U.S. citizens, 284 million.[3] You come up with an annual health care cost per citizen of roughly $4,930. That's today's number. Add a conservative 10 percent a year for two years, and the tax burden would exceed $5,000 per American just to sustain our current system.

These are fairly rough numbers, but they are accurate enough to make an important point about moving to a single-payer, government-run system. What tax source would be used to come up with $5,000 per citizen (man, woman, and child) if the government were to become the sole payer of all health care bills?

We Already Pay Higher Health Care Taxes Than the Brits Do

The good news is that the single-payer tax burden wouldn't all have to come from new taxes. It's important to note that our government already pays a major portion of our national health bill with our tax dollars. Remember that we do have a lot of government health care coverage already. In fact, we already spend more tax money buying care than the Brits do. If you add up the current costs of Medicare ($241 billion) and Medicaid ($232 billion),[4] and then add in the costs of other government programs such as the Defense Department, Veterans' Health, and other public health programs, and then add to that the costs of providing health insurance coverage for state and federal government employees, you reach a government-funded total of $630 billion. In other words, we already pay for a huge amount of care with tax money. That total tax expense for currently government-funded care, divided among our citizens, already comes to about $2,218 per citizen per year. All of those programs are now funded by our government, so we already pay that full amount with our current taxes.

The U.S. Government Is Not an Efficient Purchaser of Care

One thing that stands out immediately from these numbers is that our government is not a very efficient purchaser of health care services by world standards. We find it very telling that the cost to our government for providing health care benefits to just a portion of our population already exceeds the full per citizen government care expenditure in Great Britain. In Britain, the government spends $1,763 in tax dollars per person per year to buy universal coverage for all citizens. Our government already directly spends $2,218 per person in tax money, and that money buys care for just the old, the poor, the disabled, and the governmentally employed. To say it very clearly, we already spend a lot more in per capita tax dollars than the Brits do, and we cover only a small subset of our population with that money. They use far less money to cover everyone in the country, citizen and guest alike.

That fact has to give pause to advocates of a single-payer system for the United States. It tells us clearly that savings and efficiencies will not result automatically from having the U.S. government buy care. It is possible that there could be some administrative savings from a single-payer program. However, health care expenditures are likely to remain high in this country given our technology and cultural imperatives for all possible care.

In any case, if we factor in the current government expenditures for health care and use the $4,930 current health care cost as a base, these numbers tell us that the actual new and additional tax burden for Americans would not be $1.4 trillion, but the difference between $1.4 trillion and $630 billion—or $770 billion in new money if the person started today. On a pure per capita basis, the additional annual tax burden for every American would be $2,711. Again, this would simply be to maintain the status quo, with no allowance for inflation in health care costs, assuming we convert to a national insurance plan this year. Even in a crisis, Congress can't act that quickly. The fastest imaginable plan would take at least three years to implement.

Add in a very optimistic 10 percent inflation for three years, and that new tax number would approach $3,600 per capita. For a family of four, the additional tax burden to pay for a single-payer system in the United States would be over $14,000. That assumes no new technology and no new drugs after three years.

That's a lot of additional government spending. It's also a huge cut in people's take-home pay if the tax burden is distributed evenly to all citizens. Most of that money is now spent by employers. If people were given raises that equaled their current health care premiums and then taxed on the new wages, the total amount of our new expense would be less—but still far more than the current out-of-pocket payroll deduction levels for most consumers. Probably America is not yet ready for it, particularly if what we will inevitably get for our money is significantly rationed access to care.

A decade ago, both the Canadians and the British were bragging about the successes of their national health systems. Today, that bragging has been replaced by budget crises, cutbacks in care, and long waits for essential services. Similar stories are emerging in other countries whose health programs are run exclusively by the government. For example, the governing German Social Democratic Party called for a radical change in health care policy in 2001, replacing the current budgeted system with a market-driven system. The party called for increased competition at all levels of the health system.[5] In the most recent British elections, a hotly debated topic included voter dissatisfaction with inadequate hospital care, nonexistent specialty care, and astonishingly long waits for complex medical procedures. No one in those countries denies that major problems exist. No one wants to pay the taxes necessary to fix them.

Why do the citizens of those other countries put up with those levels of care rationing? Again, a consideration of the actuarial information in Chapter Three—that 1 percent of the population uses 30 percent of the total health care costs—can help explain the political realities of government-run health care. This is an extremely important point to understand. The government in each of those countries invests the bulk of its money on primary care, not specialty care or hospital care. Why? Look at Figure 10.1. Again, you will see that the vast majority of all citizens (voters) incur relatively low health care costs because most of their needs are met at the primary care level.

In any given year, the vast majority of British and Canadian voters are relatively healthy, so they have their perceived care needs met by the availability of local primary care doctors. Only a very small percentage of the population in any country actually need open heart surgery or hospital stays. In countries with national health insurance, some of those very sick people get that specialty level of care. Others do not. In some countries, more do. But polit-

Figure 10.1. Voting Power in the Single-Payer Health Care System

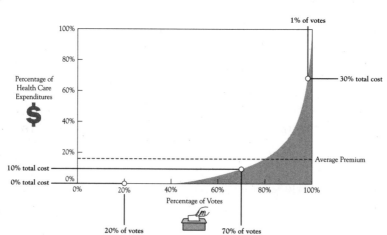

Source: Milliman USA Health Cost Guidelines—2001 Claim Probability Distributions.

ically, the ones who do not are a small percentage of the total population of voters. A cynic might note that each government in power gives regular "safety valve" speeches about planning future upgrades in specialty care. Those speeches give hope to the vast majority of healthy citizens about the future likelihood of having specialty care available when today's healthy people might actually need it. That whole process limits general anxiety and leads to a level of complaints and voter stress that is constant but politically manageable. The politicians know that dying people on the right-hand side of the continuum are probably too sick to vote and make up only a tiny voting bloc at best anyway.

In the United States, anyone on the right side of the continuum expects great care, instantly available and fully paid for. That expectation (and those costs) doesn't exist anywhere else in the world.

Germany Offers an Interesting Model

Of all national health care systems that exist in the world today, the one that might have the greatest likelihood of success in the United States is the German system. In Germany, each citizen selects membership in a health fund—an organization that collects premiums from the government and is then responsible for delivering all needed care. Some variation on that model might work in the United States if the payment levels are established to give the equivalents of vouchers to each American citizen, with the ability of each citizen to use the voucher as a payment for care in a health fund of his or her choice.

It would take a period of transition to get to that model. A marketplace that could use the vouchers would have to be created. If that sounds familiar, it should. That was the essence of the Clinton administration's managed competition model.

Although that proposal has already failed politically in this country, it might have a second chance once all other possible systems have been examined and politically rejected. The system has merit—but no political support with either consumers or policy-makers today. It sounds too "HMO-like" to be America's option of choice at this point, regardless of its merits. That could well change.

That model could be priced to create a fixed tax burden like the British or Canadian approaches. It could also be partially implemented by new laws requiring all employers to offer some form of health coverage. Done well, that approach might create quite a bit more accountability for both efficiency and quality than either of these systems.

Price Controls Are Another Option

What other government initiatives are available to Americans if we want to keep health care costs down? Price controls for care delivery might be a possibility, at least for the short term. Someone in Washington might try to set up a national fee schedule of some kind and then limit provider payments to that schedule. That would definitely help with unit prices but would have no positive impact on volume. We've already played that game once. Prior experiments with fee controls resulted in major unit volume increases. Some providers were able to maintain their overall revenue simply by providing more care procedures per patient, whether the patient needed them or not. The games of code creep and "unnecessary callbacks" have been played before. We would have to create an immense set of very detailed rules to keep caregivers from gaming the system, and then we would need some process to monitor adherence to the rules.

Regulating fees is harder than it looks. In addition to setting fixed fees for all current services, some sort of expert government panel would also have to determine fair fees for all new technologies, new equipment, new procedures, and new drugs. These are all major cost drivers today. A price-setting panel would have a huge impact on this aspect of health care. Depending on how frugally the new panel functioned, the new procedure prices might be so low as to stop development cold for most new drugs and new technology. Or if the panel's pricing favored new approaches and made new drugs and technology even more profitable, it could accelerate the transition to new and more expensive care approaches. Many providers would be motivated to perform whatever care approach generates the most revenue. The design of the system and the pricing for care would need to be thought through very carefully.

Judging from experience, the whole price control process would be complex, controversial, and extremely unpopular with most providers of care. Resistance would be fierce. Gamesmanship in care delivery would be rampant. The likelihood of short-term success would be moderate; the likelihood of long-term success would be nonexistent.

Premium Price Controls

Another government initiative that might be considered is insurance premium price controls. But because premiums are simply the arithmetic sum of the costs of care, freezing premiums without first freezing care costs would be an immediate guarantee of insurer failure and plan bankruptcy. The California utility fiasco has already shown us all the dysfunctionality and perils of capping consumer retail prices while allowing the costs to the provider of energy to fluctuate. The same thing would happen if premiums were frozen while care costs exploded. The private insurance market would collapse quickly.

Insurance premium caps could work only if the law also gave each insurer the direct right to arbitrarily cap all provider payments at whatever the unit fees would need to be for the insurers to avoid losing money. That approach would allow plans to stay in business, at least temporarily. Providers would, we believe, oppose laws giving insurers that degree of control over provider pricing.

What does that leave? What alternative approaches might work? Maybe we need an actual health policy for this country for the first time in our history. Don't reject that idea until you've taken a look at how it might work.

Our current system has its advantages. It is constantly producing miracles of care. We have more care available than anywhere else in the world. Basic levels of care could be safer and more consistent, but those same safety and inconsistency issues exist across the planet. Our current system's virtues stem in part from the fact that the marketplace rewards innovation in some exciting ways. A government-run system would find it almost impossible to continue that innovation.

So what can be done to sustain a market-based but affordable approach to care? The next chapter offers a couple of suggestions that we believe will help.

11

· ·

Where Do We Go from Here?
A Call for a National Health Strategy

We believe that the very best way of dealing with the explosion in the costs of care might be to increase the value of the care we are buying. We believe that it's time to build a national health strategy aimed at mitigating the rate of health care cost increases while significantly improving both the value and quality of care in this country. We believe that the United States should, for the first time in its history, create a clearly articulated, carefully designed, overarching national health care strategy, with goals, initiatives, products, and processes all aimed at implementing that strategy.

Our nation has never taken that kind of systematic approach to health care. Health care in this country has developed pretty much on its own. The government has never had anything even remotely resembling an overall strategy. The care system, of course, has been influenced, supported, incented, disincented, funded, and misfunded by a plethora of various unrelated government programs. But those programs have never been coordinated by anyone in any way as part of a well-thought-out national health strategy.

In more cases than we all like to remember, in fact, various government incentives and programs have worked against each other. Regional hospital overbedding, for example, resulted from major construction projects done with "free" government funds.

If we want to fix our overall system, we need to think of all American care delivery as a macrosystem, plan for it as a system, and then reward and regulate it as a system. We do not want to end up with a bureaucratic, highly regulated, government-run system, but we do want to achieve a carefully engineered, consumer-focused, market-driven health care ecosystem. To get there, we need a strategic national plan, not just a series of reactions to the unrelated business and governmental crisis of the moment.

We Americans don't particularly like government planning in most areas of our lives. Unfortunately, because the health care delivery and financing system is now so complex and has so many parts, anything less than a comprehensive macrostrategy will probably not have sufficient impact to create a meaningful solution for either health care costs or health care quality problems.

We believe that a true national strategy would have seven key elements. We believe that as part of a true national strategy, seven major initiatives are needed (each is discussed in detail in the next seven chapters):

- Initiative One should improve quality of care and patient safety.

- Initiative Two should address consumer choices, behaviors, and incentives, creating an improved market model for both buying and selling health care.

- Initiative Three should improve population health.

- Initiative Four should prevent monopolistic and other anticompetitive behaviors.

- Initiative Five should create a workable framework for dealing with the uninsured.

- Initiative Six, to make sure miracles keep happening, should result in providing adequate support to the health care delivery system by funding training, med-

ical education, medical research, a resupply of the
health care workforce, and a reengineering of actual
health care delivery, particularly in hospital settings.

- Initiative Seven creates an underpinning for the entire
cost, value, and quality agenda: the creation of an automated medical record that will give the doctor and patient in the exam room all of the information needed
to provide best care efficiently and consistently. The
use of that system is embedded in each of the other
objectives.

As we discuss each of these major policy agendas, it's important
to state clearly that we believe that none of the resultant initiatives
would or should result in a government-run care system. All would
instead significantly strengthen a competitive marketplace focused
on the patient and health care consumer. Done well, none would
result in rationing. All would strongly encourage consumer choice.
None would result in a significantly greater U.S. tax burden. All
would make care more affordable.

President Clinton, in his early days in office, attempted to reform
the health care system by changing the market dynamic of health
insurance coverage. His plan had merit in a number of important
areas, but it created at least a sense of excessive direct government
involvement in care. Even worse, his plan wasn't explainable to
the general population. It was too complex. The labyrinth intrica-
cies of the plan delighted and activated federal policy wonks, but
they made little or no sense to the American public.

Americans don't want unnecessary complexity. Americans want
safe care, accessible care, and choices about their care. Americans
want local accountability for their care. Americans want an adequate supply of doctors, nurses, pharmacists, and technicians so that
care is available when needed. At this stage of our history, Americans also want affordable care.

An understandable health care policy that moves in those directions has a chance of success, particularly if it relies on market forces for its implementation. That's the approach suggested by these seven policy agendas. Some are possible now, without government intervention, if enlightened buyers finally begin to take advantage of their natural market leverage and act strategically. Others will require government action. All deserve our consideration. It's time to have a plan for the future of health care in this country.

So how would the seven initiatives actually work? Let's start with safety and quality.

12

. . . .

Patients Deserve Safe Care

The health care delivery nonsystem in the United States performs miracles every day. Highly skilled caregivers deliver care
that is the best in the world. If your heart fails and you need a transplant, there is no better place in the world to be.

That does not mean that our approach to care is perfect. In
truth, major elements of our care nonsystem deliver less than optimal care. For many patients, care is actually unsafe. For other patients, it is imperfect, flawed, and inconsistent. We don't take
advantage of the full array of medical science and medical wisdom
already available to us to make sure that every heart attack victim
receives best follow-up care or that every person with diabetes receives the care necessary to avoid ugly and crippling complications.
The levels of inconsistency in care delivery that define our current
nonsystem of care ought to be unacceptable to all participants in
the care process: patients, caregivers, payers, and policymakers.

It's time to incent, encourage, and support a whole new systematic approach to the delivery of care. We need both to know what
the best care practices are for any condition and how to communicate those best practices to all caregivers and patients. We need to
know what kinds of accidents are killing people in hospitals, and
we need systematic programs to prevent those accidents. We need
to know which teams of caregivers perform better at preventing second heart attacks, avoiding preterm births, delivering appropriate

diabetic care, and delivering optimal care to asthmatics. Patients need that kind of information. So do the people who actually deliver care.

This is not an academic argument. It makes a real difference in the lives of millions of individuals. When the right care can cut congestive heart failure crisis by nearly 60 percent, we, as patients, need to know which doctors and care systems are providing that care and achieving those goals. We need mechanisms to communicate that right care to all relevant caregivers, and patients deserve to know both what those best practices are and how well their own caregivers do in following them.

Right now, selecting caregivers is simply a game of chance for far too many Americans. It's pure luck if you are diabetic and end up with a doctor or medical group that actually meets minimal American Diabetes Association care standards. (Two-thirds of America's doctors currently do not meet those standards.) It's luck if your doctor knows and uses the best approach to preventing a second heart attack. (One-third of doctors do not meet those standards.) It's luck if your local emergency system is fully up to speed on the best immediate treatments of your stroke.

There has been a relatively small amount of publicity about the treatment of stroke. The condition is relatively rare but can be extremely serious. The way patients are treated can make a huge difference for the rest of their life. The differences in care outcomes for stroke patients are immense. For certain kinds of strokes, patients who get the right treatment immediately have an 80 percent chance of excellent recovery. Patients who don't get the right clot dissolvers within two hours of a major stroke have an almost 80 percent chance of being permanently damaged, and in many cases, seriously crippled for life. Think of the alternatives: crippled for life or fully functional. This is a major patient safety issue. It's one that can be remedied. Medical team and emergency room performance in those cases can be measured. Consistent best care can be encouraged. As in many other health situations, it is also important to point out that the "best care" relative to breaking up stroke clots also slightly increases the chance of excess bleeding and will have an adverse impact on some patients. It's a matter of statistics and rational decision making in a systematic way.

Which approach would you prefer if you had a stroke? The answer is obvious: the statistically valid best chance of a good outcome. But do you, right now, have any idea about what kind of care you'd get today if you personally were having a stroke?

That's the kind of information that is needed to create a care system that is both consistent and focused on constantly improving both value and results. That's the kind of information we don't have because no one in the marketplace is currently asking for it or demanding that care systems improve both value and results in those kinds of categories of care.

Buyers have been at a huge disadvantage when it comes to health care quality and value. Any manufacturer can tell you with great precision exactly what the specifications and quality standards are for any piece of equipment they purchase. The quality definition for new screws, wines, or doorknobs is precise and rigorous. By contrast, when those same manufacturers buy health care for their employees, there have been only a few standards even available, and very little emphasis placed on using even those standards in actually buying care or selecting caregivers.

It's time for buyers to evolve into more sophisticated purchasing mechanisms. How can that be done? By taking advantage of some existing quality standards and insisting on the development of others.

The American Diabetes Association Pioneered Accountability

The American Diabetes Association took a huge step in this direction four years ago with a revolutionary approach. It used a panel of the most respected caregivers, scientists, and researchers to develop a set of basic care standards for doctors to follow with their

162 EPIDEMIC OF CARE

diabetic patients. If doctors fully follow these standards, they have the potential to detect complications early and reduce major complications such as amputations, blindness, and kidney failure by more than 50 percent. Fifty percent fewer blind people. Fifty percent fewer patients with kidney failure. These are huge steps forward.

That ADA program represented the first attempt by a medical specialty group in the United States to build scientifically sound, evidence-based care protocols for people with a particular disease. The ADA then took the next important step and used a carefully designed screening process to identify which caregivers were meeting standards. It now publicly recognizes those caregivers and has recently teamed up with the National Committee for Quality Assurance (NCQA) to advance this groundbreaking program.

Unfortunately, very few people in positions of authority or influence understand the importance of the ADA/NCQA program. Buyers don't even look at it when they select health care plans. Congress should have celebrated that program. They ignored it. So did the media. The American news media utterly failed to see how important that program was. The general public therefore knows nothing about the ADA's extraordinary work.

Why was the program ignored? Because the local media simply do not understand how inconsistent most diabetic care actually is or how many people go blind, lose limbs, go into kidney failure, or die of a heart attack because their diabetes is inadequately treated. Those stories aren't told, so a program that fixes those problems isn't perceived to have any value. No one appreciates solutions unless they have first appreciated the problem.

As a result, absolutely no public pressure is being put on less-than-effective caregivers to improve their care. That is a shame. It's a great program. The ADA itself deserves major recognition for being a pioneer—a courageous, enlightened pioneer—in making care both better and more accountable. We call the ADA courageous because it implemented its provider recognition program in the face of significant resistance from a sizable subset of caregivers who did not particularly want to be measured.

That means some diabetes patients will suffer much more than they need to. It also means many health care dollars will be wasted. Unaccountable, inconsistent, inferior care costs a lot of money. Bad care outcomes cost a lot of money. Unnecessary heart attacks, unnecessary CHF crisis, and avoidable preterm births are all very bad care that also cost a lot of money. Having people permanently and unnecessarily crippled by strokes is expensive. As a society, we are paying top dollar for what is too often wasteful, dangerous, and inconsistent care.

That's particularly frustrating because we know from experience in a number of settings that systematic use of medical best practices can significantly improve care and, in a great many cases, also save money. It generally costs significantly less to do care right. It costs a lot less, for example, to prevent a preterm birth than it does to spend upwards of $500,000 on that baby's first hospital stay.

How can best practices be introduced more broadly into care delivery across the nation? The largest and best care systems are already putting programs in place to identify best practices and roll them out systematically. Recent analyses of data provided by Hewitt Associates, NCQA, and Healthy People 2010 show distinctly better performance on a wide range of quality measures for group practice–based plans compared with plans primarily using single physician practices.[1] Most physicians, however, do not practice in those large, multispecialty groups with enough resources to do their own research into best practices. For those nongroup practitioners, some other process needs to happen. One good approach might be to have other specialty organizations follow the ADA's lead and identify specific standards of care built around the best current medical science to systematically improve care outcomes. Why doesn't the American Neurological Society (ANS) have an evidence-based standard of best care for emergency stroke victims? Why doesn't it have both an up-to-date protocol for emergency stroke care and a process to review that protocol every three months to make sure it's still the best? Why doesn't it follow the ADA lead and let us all know which stroke response teams are safest and which are inadvertently and unintentionally dooming far too many patients to a lifetime of dysfunctionality and disability?

Public policy in this country should encourage and support both the development of those best practices and the systematic distribution of that information to all American doctors.

There are probably 20,000 doctors in this country who treat strokes. There are probably 5,000 emergency rooms that treat stroke crisis.[2] They need a consistent approach. How can all 20,000 physicians and all 5,000 ERs keep up on the latest developments in early stroke reaction? They can't, but a national specialty association such as the ANS can. The associations for other specialties should do the same. National public policy and national funds in this country should support both the development of these evidence-based, outcomes-focused best practices and the systematic distribution of that information to all American doctors, other caregivers, hospitals, and patients. The government should strongly support that process. And then we as a nation need a distribution mechanism to get that information to every relevant caregiver, care team, ER, and patient.

Targeted Internet Communications Can Get Best Practices to All Relevant Physicians

For the first time in history, we have a mechanism in place that can accomplish that massive, customized, highly targeted information-sharing goal with a high level of efficiency. That mechanism is the Internet. Distribution of truly current information about medical best practices has always been a real challenge. Doctors are often too busy to read about every available scientific development, and the best doctors tend to be very busy. Printed medical journals are seen by only a subset of caregivers. We need a much better way of getting key new information to our caregivers. This is particularly true when different types of caregivers are all relevant to the care of a given condition or patient. Every specialty has its own journals, seminars, and publications. Those publications have to be targeted at particular subsets of caregivers. Printed information about issues that cross the lines between specialties or between hospitals and physicians often doesn't exist. Even if it did exist, it would have to be distributed individually through separate publications for each category of caregiver.

That whole process of keeping doctors current through the equivalent of magazine articles has been extremely slow, entirely undependable, and woefully inadequate. We have long needed better mechanisms for distributing that kind of information. Direct mail to specific caregivers on some key issues might have been possible, but the logistics of that process made even that limited effort functionally undoable. If there are 30,000 cardiologists, who would make the mailing? Who would keep the mailing list accurate? Who would pay for the postage? It's easy to see why the current method of information distribution about newly discovered best practices has not been as consistent or thorough as patients might hope.

To deal with that problem, we can use the Internet.

The Internet provides a wonderful new set of highly customizable communication tools that will let us overcome almost all of the historic communication barriers for the distribution of new medical science.

The first challenge is to have a source for that key medical information that is current, state of the art, and entirely credible. The second challenge is to have Internet addresses for all of the physicians who might be relevant to any major new development in care. Both tasks are major, but both can be done.

The availability of the Internet as a care improvement communication tool has the potential to transform the way care is delivered in the United States for those physicians who are not part of large multispecialty group practices.

If major announcements about significant research findings and care effectiveness studies are appropriately flagged, they could be sent directly to every targeted recipient. Doctors and other caregivers would then have an easy way of being current. Patients would benefit. And some progress would be made.

Major Progress Will Require Automated Decision Support Tools

Those communication and process improvement levels are all, at best, interim stages. Real improvement in the quality and consistency of care will require the use of automated medical records that give doctors and patients full information about care and care systems right in the exam room.

Ultimately, as medical practitioners increasingly use automated medical record systems, the very best science-based medical practice protocols can be embedded in those systems to make the information available to each caregiver at the optimal time. When a doctor treats a patient and calls up the patient's screen right in the exam room, that's a great opportunity to remind the doctor of what his or her peers believe is the best protocol for that patient.

Large multispecialty group practices will have an initial advantage over the independent, solo practice doctors, because the larger practices are much more likely to have an automated medical record support structure in place.

In traditional American medicine, all information about the care delivered to patients resides on paper records kept physically in each physician's office. Those records are not integrated with each other. A patient who sees five different doctors over the course of a year generally will have five separate medical records. Doctors who see the patient in one setting generally do not have access to information about that patient that exists in another setting.

That's one of the reasons that so many patients end up with a prescription for medications that actually create dangerous health problems when combined with other prescriptions given by other physicians. Typically, no one has enough information to coordinate that whole process well.

By contrast, when that traditional paper-based medical record approach is replaced by an automated, computerized medical record, with all available information for any given patient, the ability of the caregiver to deliver better care is significantly enhanced. When the doctor in the exam room can quickly scan all test results, diagnoses, and treatments for a given patient for the past several years, treatment decisions are easier, and care is more effective.

If the computer system also makes available information about the best treatment options for the patient's current disease, then the care process is further enhanced. Every other profession makes use of computers to perform these kinds of services. Medicine will soon follow. In that setting, the likelihood of inconsistent care will diminish, and the likelihood of best care will be enhanced.

Once best practice guidelines are in place, they should be accessible to the public as well, so America's patients can know what the best current treatments are for their conditions.

Guidelines, Not Rules, for Best Care

While we strongly support disseminating best care protocols, we do not mean to suggest that America should move to cookie-cutter medicine. Nor do we believe that anyone should impose absolute rules for any kind of care. Far from it. It is critically important that the best practice communications be seen as guidelines, not rules. It is the individual doctor treating each individual patient who needs to make the actual treatment decisions. Any of a myriad of factors could cause an excellent, highly skilled doctor to vary care from even the best care guidelines. Comorbidities, for example, could cause alternative decisions about care; so might allergies or psychological problems or even financial or sociological issues. These are factors that could not be known to the protocol developers. Doctors in consultation with their patients need to be in control of care.

What matters is that variances in treatment approaches are due to conscious medical decision making, not just a lack of information on the part of the doctor about current best science for any given condition.

We are not recommending cookbook medicine, but even the best cooks often consult cookbooks. When, as discussed in Chapter Two, 135 doctors, each working independently, deliver eighty-two different treatments to one patient, then giving some current scientific information to about 80 of those physicians might be in their patient's best interest.

Web clearinghouses for protocols and best practices already exist. All payers, all policyholders, and all citizens should urge doctors to use them. The federal government should support mechanisms for the targeted distribution of that knowledge.

Local Best Practice Consortiums Can Succeed Now

We don't have to wait for the government or for national specialty organizations to act in order to benefit locally from the systematic application of medical best practices. Large multispecialty group practices should work hard now to identify best practices and communicate them to the group members. The ability to do that kind of care improvement is one of the major advantages of the group practice.

We've proven in Minnesota that it is also possible for local doctors to get together to develop and use evidence-based medicine and best practice protocols. Other areas of the country might want to look at the successful pioneering program of the Institute for Clinical Systems Improvement in Minnesota (ICSI).

ICSI created a community consortium made up of the best medical minds in Minnesota. Physicians from Mayo Clinic, HealthPartners Medical Group, Park Nicollet Health Services, and two dozen other local medical groups get together on a regular basis to figure out medical best practices for selected conditions. The protocols are then used to guide care in the community. To date, ICSI has developed protocols for more than fifty conditions, ranging from simple cystitis (bladder infection) to heart attack follow-up.[3] It is important to point out that the program is a cooperative medical collaborative, led and governed by local physicians. Funding for ICSI's first seven years came exclusively from HealthPartners. HealthPartners is a consumer-owned, consumer-governed health plan. Its focus is on improving care for consumers, so it has been willing to invest money in care improvement programs at a relatively high level. The program for care improvement has been a success. Now all local payers in Minnesota (Blue Cross and Blue Shield of Minnesota, PreferredOne, UCare, Metropolitan Health Plan, and the others) contribute to support the program. Independent doctors run it. Payers fund it. Patients get better care.

Care is better because all parties are better off when care for all major conditions is systematically built around the best medical science. In the ICSI model, physicians determine best care. All payers then agree to support best care, as defined by the doctors. Each local health plan can then add value by paying and by measuring relative caregiver performance in their networks in the context of ICSI protocols.

ICSI not only builds medical protocols; it also updates them every twelve to eighteen months. Medical science changes, so ICSI has a process in place to keep up. Once the protocols are developed or revised, they are moved out to the medical community directly by ICSI and indirectly by the health plans.

ICSI protocols are available to all doctors on the Web and in hard copy. The guidelines are also on the National Guideline Clearinghouse Web site, sponsored by the Agency for Healthcare Research and Quality. They have been embedded in several local automated medical record systems and help guide performance in this way as well.

Patients Also Need Access to Current Medical Guidelines

The ICSI protocols are also available to all Minnesota patients on the Web. Patients may go to the Web site to learn how the best doctors in the state believe their condition should be handled.

Consumers benefit very directly. Care has measurably improved. As one example, beta blocker follow-up after a heart attack has reached 98 percent at HealthPartners in large part due to ICSI leadership.[4] That performance is 50 percent higher than national averages.

At Kaiser Permanente, the Care Management Institute (CMI) performs a similar function and achieves similar exceptional results. The Kaiser Permanente patients are now at a 97 percent level for beta blocker follow-up, for example. Diabetic care within the Permanente Medical Group achieves some of the highest scores in the nation. These successes are not accidental.[5]

Payers Need to Reward the Use of Protocols

ICSI-like organizations could and should be started in many other communities. Buyers should work to encourage the health plans they use to be involved in ICSI-like consortiums, particularly in communities where a CMI-like effect isn't available. If ICSI or CMI-like structures aren't available, communities can go to the ICSI Web site and borrow the protocols. ICSI makes them available to all users.

The protocols aren't the biggest challenge. The biggest challenge is creating a consortium of physicians and payers who agree that protocols are important. Recently, twenty or so of the nation's largest and best multispecialty group practices have united to form the Council of Accountable Group Practices, a nonprofit group dedicated to using their leadership to further the national quality improvement agenda. It is gratifying to see this sort of long-needed proactive effort from the physician practice community.

A comparable level of reform will not happen in most communities until and unless the buyers and payers insist that their health plans use a best care system. Payers need to reward use of protocols by plans and providers. From a market perspective, employers could be the key. Employers have great economic leverage, but really haven't had any way of using that leverage to improve the quality of care. That's not the buyers' fault; it's hard to demand a nonexistent feature or program. Now that ICSI exists, employers should ask their local health plans to prove they are encouraging and rewarding similar protocol use by the plan's care network and providers.

Buyers Need Plan Data; Patients Need Doctor Data

One measure of comparative overall plan performance that many employers currently use are the HEDIS reports, made available by the NCQA. These reports show overall plan provider network performance relative to a dozen areas, including diabetes follow-up and beta blocker use. For those areas, buyers can now track improvement in plan performance from year to year.

These reports, however, are not in themselves sufficient to let employers know whether care protocols are being used in many other important areas, such as hypertension follow-up and stroke complication prevention. For those areas, buyers should ask plans and medical groups directly what quality improvement activities are under way.

The HEDIS reports have been under attack by some people who say that the reports in their current form are irrelevant to most consumers. That is, in fact, true. When HEDIS shows comparative data between various local and national health plans in follow-up care for a condition like diabetes, that information is most relevant at the macro plan level. It shows average performance for the entire care network used by a plan. Macrolevel data are, of course, very useful to employers because they tell employers whether each plan is making overall improvements in key areas of care.

These same reports are much less useful to individual patients and consumers because HEDIS does not now report performance at the individual provider or medical group level. HEDIS reports only aggregate, planwide data. Consumers, of course, get care from individual doctors and from medical groups, not from large, artificially aggregated networks of doctors.

Current HEDIS data for any single plan are too melded for consumer use if it involves multiple, unrelated medical practices. An average planwide C-section rate of 15 per 100 births, for example, doesn't tell consumers that one OB group in the plan network has a C-section rate of 10 while the group next door has a C-section rate of 30. These numbers indicate a major difference in caregiver performance and philosophy. As a patient, you know something useful when you compare 10 to 30. But an average planwide number of 15 doesn't help in the least when you're looking for a doctor to deliver your baby.

This is not to say that aggregate, planwide data are not useful. They very much are. Buyers should want to know if a health plan is making overall improvements across its entire provider network. Buyers pick entire plans for their employees, not individual doctors.

If a plan, overall, has dropped its C-section rate from 19 to 15 over two years, that's very useful information to the buyer. It says that the plan is working on that particular quality issue and therefore influencing provider behavior. Those data help employers pick plans but do not help individual patients pick individual physicians. HEDIS is, as it is usually now set up, a buyer tool rather than a patient tool. It can, however, be modified by health plans to serve as a patient tool also. In Minnesota, HealthPartners went to the next step and set up an Internet reporting system for patients showing actual HEDIS performance by each local care team and care system. It can be done for most measurements.

The HealthPartners Web site tells patients, for example, how each local care team treating people with diabetes does on improving blood sugar levels for their patients. This more detailed reporting process gives consumers useful information that can help them choose the best local care team.

Performance Reporting Improves Care

A second benefit of measuring individual providers, medical groups, and care teams is that care often improves significantly when provider performance is publicly reported.

All doctors are A students. When credible comparable measurements show lower-than-A performance, the natural tendency of almost all physicians is to improve performance. So when a given physician or care team learns it has earned a C or D grade compared to other local caregivers, the immediate response is almost always to improve performance. That response benefits patients and caregivers alike.

As time goes on, it will be possible to provide consumers with an increasingly sophisticated set of comparative reports about care team performance. Those reports can help in a number of areas. Smart buyers should be requiring their plans to provide that information on a regular basis. Check the Minnesota Web site (www.healthpartners. com) to see what's possible.

The Limits of Individual Provider Data

The usefulness and scope of individual provider performance reports are inherently limited by some very basic laws of statistics and mathematical measurement. Most providers do not have enough patients with some diseases for reports about any given doctor's outcomes for those particular diseases to be statistically relevant. There are, of course, exceptions. It can be statistically relevant if all patients of a given doctor with a given disease die quickly. The response to that particular piece of information should be an immediate peer-based or plan-based quality review, however, and not an annually updated Internet report.

We believe patients should have comparative performance data, but we also strongly believe that patients should not choose or reject their doctors based on statistically irrelevant reports. It would, in fact, be grossly irresponsible to produce provider performance reports that influenced and guided consumer behavior but were statistically unsound.

The good news is that a fair number of important procedures and measurements are normally performed in sufficiently high volume to present statistically significant data. C-sections by OB group, for example, are done with enough frequency to be measurable, re-portable, and comparable. Blood sugar management levels also, we believe, provide valid comparative information about doctors who treat a number of people with diabetes.

Premature birth is a much rarer event. Although premature births have a huge impact on people's lives and create major cost consequences, they usually don't happen often enough to create sta-tistically meaningful data for any single small OB group or any in-dividual obstetrician. The data are relevant for large OB groups and relevant on a planwide basis, but not statistically credible for indi-vidual doctors (unless the numbers for a given doctor are so outra-geous that they trigger a plan quality review process).

We know that reporting preterm birthrates by individual physi-cians on the Web would result in the display of entirely unreliable data, making some physicians look undeservedly good and others undeservedly bad relative to their actual care performance. If we gave consumers that outcome information on the Web, we would be entirely unfair. It would be reporting random statistical fluctua-tions, not medical performance.

When Outcomes Aren't Statistically Valid, Track Process

So how do we know which doctors are doing a good job in pre-venting preterm birth? It's obviously an important issue. The an-swer is to measure process, not outcomes when outcomes aren't available or statistically valid. We want to know who is following medical best practices for these patients.

When tracking outcomes is statistically misleading, we can still track physician compliance with protocols. There are, we now know, measurable process steps that indicate whether a given OB group is performing well on the care approaches necessary for avoiding preterm births. We can measure whether risk screenings are being done. We can track whether high-risk mothers are being identified. We can track whether those mothers are being helped. We can, in other words, track certain key process indicators and then report whether physicians are, in fact, working systematically to prevent preterm births. That's a valid way of tracking performance because we know that prevention processes, in the aggregate, reduce those births.

The whole process needs to take measurements at the level where measurements are both valid and useful. As a rule, we've learned over time that performance for some types of care can be measured at the care team level as actual outcomes (second heart attacks, for example), while for other types of care, performance can be determined only using process measurements (diabetic foot checks, for example).

A sophisticated reporting system will use both types of reporting. It's time for America to start using such sophisticated reporting so patients can begin to see which care providers are best for safe and effective care. It's time for health plans to begin implementing these kinds of sophisticated measurements. None of this will happen, however, until the market recognizes the value of performance reporting and rewards it.

Systematic Review of Care Outcomes Can Reap Quick Awards

Care improvement is necessary if we are going to achieve full value from our health care dollar. Systematic care improvement is also necessary if we are going to make care as safe as it ought to be.

One fascinating study done by Kaiser Permanente in its Colorado Region looked at the issue of mammography accuracy. The head of the radiology department decided to review how well each radiologist in the department was doing in reading the images that indicated whether a given woman had a breast lump that might be cancerous. The study showed a significant variation in the physicians' skill set in picking out those lumps at a very early stage, when the cancers are most treatable.

In part, the study identified women with Stage Two, Three, or Four breast cancer and looked back at mammograms taken of those women earlier to see if a second set of medical eyes could have detected the cancers a year earlier at Stage One. It turned out that the skill levels were different in that regard. The medical group decided to take a couple of different approaches to the situation. Some physicians were retrained. Others were assigned to reading other kinds of X rays and electronic images.

In a relatively short time, the number of cancers not detected until a later stage dropped from 14 percent to 6 percent. Dozens of lives have been saved. That happened even though the doctors reading the mammograms were all trained radiologists. In the non–Kaiser Permanente world, those X rays are often read by internists and family practitioners with much lower levels of training. Some of those independent physicians do a superb job. Others do not. If it was your mammogram, wouldn't you like a system in place to track caregiver accuracy in that area? Right now, that system exists only in one place.

Systematic improvements in care are possible. They are, in fact, needed. But in today's health care marketplace, they are not rewarded.

Why Haven't Buyers Rewarded Quality Care?

Employers and government agencies have not been particularly demanding buyers up to this point when it comes to care quality. This has been due, in large part, to the fact that the science of caregiver performance measurement is still in its embryonic stages. Buyers haven't really had an array of available measurement options for most categories of care, so they haven't insisted on provider measurement. Up to now, it has not been common practice in this country for employers to use quality measures as they make decisions about which plans to use for their employees. That makes perfect sense when quality measures are either nonexistent or too rudimentary to be meaningful.

However, even in cases where measurements have existed, a great many buyers have tended not to use them, for several reasons. Some employers tell us that they believe that all care is equal and all plans, in the end, provide roughly the same quality care. For those buyers, the current set of quality reports is a nonissue.

Other employers choose their plan based solely on price and network location and ignore the quality reports that are available because that's how some benefit managers see their assignment. No benefit manager in the country, or his or her corporate chief financial or chief executive officer, has ever been fired for not choosing the HMO with the best HEDIS scores for patients with diabetes, but many benefit managers have been fired for offering HMOs whose premiums were, in the opinion of the benefit manager's boss, too high. The top executives typically hold benefit managers accountable for cost and, sometimes, employee satisfaction levels but not the quality of a plan's care or relative success in the prevention of disease or disease complications.

Guess where the benefit managers' usual priorities lie? Their bosses want them to make an economic decision. So they generally do.

We believe that should, and will, change.

Healthy Employees Are on the Job

A strong economic case can be made for quality. Healthy employees are on the job. Employees with healthy children take fewer personal days or "sick" days. Better care also saves money on recovery time, getting workers (and parents) back to work more quickly.

Unfortunately, up to now, no one has done a good job of explaining to benefit managers or their bosses why quality measurements in those areas make practical sense. No one shows how better-quality care in most cases saves money. Employers tend to make business decisions, not philosophical or ideological decisions, and the business case for using comparative provider performance data has not been well made.

That's a shame, because that data are both valuable and available. If more providers help women avoid premature births, employers can save large sums of money *and* keep parents on the job. If more providers help people avoid clinical depression, employers save significant amounts of money in care dollars and even more money by having effective, productive, functional, on-the-job workers.

It's a chicken-and-egg situation at this point. Many plans will not invest any more in quality measurements if buyers won't use them. Buyers won't ever see those data or those expanded quality programs if plans don't produce them.

It is a win-win business case for plans to produce the data and for buyers to use those data and reward better outcomes. We know that when the data are produced and used well, provider performance improves, care is better, consumers make better choices, and employers save money.

Although most buyers still don't appreciate care quality reporting systems, a growing number are taking note. Increasingly, for the best health plans, quality programs break premium ties in their favor when employers are choosing between the highest-quality plans and other plans.

As more employers come to understand the value of performance reporting and decide to buy coverage from plans that use it, we believe market forces can quickly restructure and reform health care.

Our National Policy Should Focus on Best Practices

When study after study shows immense differences in care patterns, market to market and provider to provider, it seems entirely illogical that buyers and health care policymakers have managed to ignore those data rather than use them to improve care.

In any case, care can be improved. That's been proven. Care protocols can be developed. It has been done. Provider compliance with important protocols can be tracked and reported. It has been done. Outcomes can be measured. That also has been done. The overall delivery system can, in fact, be made better and more accountable. It would be a shame to do any less.

The government role in that process can be critical. The government, as a payer, needs to encourage and reward quality care. At the same time, it needs to let specific care approaches be developed by the market. If the government puts in place a cumbersome, bureaucratic process that develops lowest-common-denominator care protocols and then locks them rigidly into place, impervious to new medical science, then the government will actually be working against quality improvement.

Some people do, however, recommend that the government perform at that micromanagement level, perhaps using "expert panels" to dictate best practices and then serve as the universal definer of all data.

The government should fund practical research into issues like hospital safety or operational implementation of medical protocols. A more useful role for the government might be to fund the communication systems that transmit the best protocols to all relevant caregivers. The government should also fund practical research into issues like hospital safety or operational implementation of medical protocols.

Hospitals would benefit immensely from grants that could be used only to put in place the kinds of systems that help ensure patient safety. In some instances, the rate of hospital-based fatal accidents could be cut by more than half if hospitals simply automated their internal care ordering process. Most hospitals can't afford these new systems on their own. Government money to subsidize these systems would make America's hospitals safer very quickly. That clearly should be part of our national health care policy.

Medical groups and medical societies also would benefit from research dollars to investigate what specific steps are needed for the successful dissemination of medical best practice protocols and to develop means of measuring the outcomes of that care. If the government commits adequate money to these efforts, the impact could be both fast and huge.

The government could also use its immense leverage as a buyer to insist on certain levels of reporting and protocol compliance for the plans and providers it uses. Rather than develop a set preterm birth protocol, the government, as a buyer, could insist that each plan it uses build or buy these types of protocols and then use them for patients. There is a fine line between being a smart buyer and a micromanager. The government needs to stay on the right side of that line.

In any case, we need to make care safer and better for all of our citizens. We can't continue to let massive levels of inconsistencies stand between patients and best care. Creating consistently safe care should be a major focus of our new national health policy. Systematic approaches to care delivery should be recognized, saluted, encouraged, and rewarded, or we will continue to have inconsistent follow-up care for people with diabetes and misread mammograms for women with breast cancer.

We spend too much money on care for that level of quality to be the American standard.

. . . .

13

401(k) Equivalent Choices in Health Care

As employers look at the surge in health care costs, a significant number have begun to wonder whether they could move away from their traditional support for a defined set of health care benefits to a new model of health care financing based on defined contribution levels.

Employers have already made that move relative to pension plans. Most U.S. employers no longer offer defined-benefit pension plans, where the employer guarantees a preset level of pension benefits for the full life of the retired worker. Instead, most employers now offer a 401(k) or 403(b) pension plan approach, where the employer gives each worker a fixed amount of money each month. Employees then invest that money in their own pension plan. In that setting, each worker is given a set of carefully selected investment opportunities and can make decisions about how to invest the monthly money.

In a defined-contribution model, the employer is off the financial hook once the monthly contribution is made to the worker. In the defined-benefit model, the employer remains on the hook for the life of the worker, accountable for creating and maintaining dedicated investment reserves that are adequate to fund the promised benefits permanently.

The recent stock market devaluation made the advantage of that model to employers extremely clear. Quite a few businesses would have been financially impaired over the past year or so had they been required to bring pension plan reserves up to full funding levels necessary to guarantee full payouts. But for many workers who had their personal pensions tied to the 401(k) investments, the stock market drop was a disaster.

Quite a few employers are now wondering whether a similar model of "defined-contribution financing" is available for health care, that is, a model that gives each employee a fixed amount of money every month and then lets each worker make individual health care coverage decisions. That model could, at least theoretically, cap employer expenses while giving employees incentives to make cost-conscious decisions about their benefit packages and care.

Some insurance vendors, looking to take advantage of that emerging buyer interest in defined-contribution plans, have offered products that are designed around some variation of defined contribution.

Will those products be the future of American health care? Can they help employers control health care costs? Some might help. Others could do considerable damage to a significant number of people. The answer depends on the product design and the funding philosophy.

It makes sense, in the context of this book, to look at a couple of the approaches that are being widely considered or at least discussed.

Medical Savings Accounts

One product variation that has created quite a bit of conversation and some political support has been a benefit design referred to as medical savings accounts (MSAs). A standard MSA package gives each worker between $500 and $1,000 in upfront, discretionary money to spend on health care. That money can be spent only on a defined set of benefits. Once the $500 or $1,000 is spent, the typical plan subjects the worker to a significant deductible—an annual direct expense to the worker of $1,000 to $3,000—depending on the plan. In other words, once the worker has spent the $500 in cash from the "savings account," the next $1,000 in expenses comes out of the worker's own pocket.

Once the $1,000 in out-of-pocket money is gone, an insurance-like benefit level kicks in and pays for additional expenses that the worker might have. The theory is that workers will be better purchasers of health care services if the first $500 spent is "free" benefit money that they totally control and the next $1,000 is money that comes directly out of their own pocket.

Proponents of that approach say that the workers will, given that benefit package, ask for lower-cost drugs and negotiate lower provider fees when they need care. Some initial studies do seem to show lower health care costs for people with that type of plan.

To appreciate the full impact of that type of benefit configuration fully, see Figure 13.1, which revisits the concept of Figure 3.1. Remember that 70 percent of the people in any given group usually create only 10 percent of the costs. Twenty percent of the people generate no costs. At the other extreme, 1 percent of the group creates 30 percent of the costs. So if an MSA product is offered to a group of people alongside a full level of benefits, which people will select the MSA as their option: the people on the left side of the continuum or the people on the right?

Obviously, the zero users on the left side of the continuum will see a direct benefit from taking the MSA benefit and receiving $500 to $1,000 in spendable money. (Some of the MSA plans expand benefit definitions to include therapeutic massages or even cosmetic procedures.)

In any case, if the MSA premium is cheaper than the full benefit package, there's little risk for someone on the left side of the continuum to pick the MSA product. They're not expecting any expenses anyway. Someone with cancer, diabetes, AIDS, hypertension, or congestive heart failure would have to be a bit silly to select an MSA product over a full benefit package. People on the high-cost right side of the cost continuum would tend to select their own doctors and full benefits.

Figure 13.1. Why MSAs Alone Will Not Solve Health Care Costs

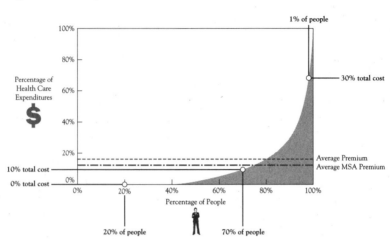

Source: Milliman USA Health Cost Guidelines—2001 Claim Probability Distributions.

A HealthPartners internal study showed that the people who left its clinics and moved to an MSA product (when offered) averaged less than half as much money in care in the year prior to the MSA plan being offered. They had the same average age as the people who stayed with the traditional plan, but much different patterns of preselection care. That makes both logical and intuitive sense.

If you look at the cost continuum chart (Figure 13.1), you will see that the dotted line represents the average cost level of the group. The line, then, is the premium needed for the group. If, for example, 10 percent of the group have no health care costs and choose to leave the group for MSA coverage, the new average premium need is 10 percent higher for the people who keep their full benefit coverage.

What about the contention that people with an MSA product make better and cheaper care choices? That's very likely true—but statistically irrelevant. If the 70 percent of the population who uses 10 percent of the care buy MSA coverage and become 10 percent more efficient, that cuts the total cost of care by 1 percent, not exactly a silver bullet.

And in the real world, what is the likelihood that an MSA enrollee who has been just diagnosed with a serious cancer is going to start negotiating treatment fees with his or her oncologist or that a heart attack victim will issue a request for proposal (RFP) while having a heart attack? Even if someone does decide to issue an RFP or negotiate physician or hospital fees, how will that person know if he or she has negotiated a good fee? If HMOs get a 20 percent discount and an MSA patient negotiates a 10 percent discount, the 10 percent discount may feel good, but it's not optimal purchasing.

People do price-shop for cosmetic surgery. That happens all the time in nonemergency settings where all prices are clearly posted. People tend not to quibble, however, on prices with the oncologist who has just diagnosed your personal cancer and is standing between you and death's door.

This isn't to say that MSAs don't have their place. For smaller groups of healthy people, they can offer a nice benefit. But as a way of solving the overall health care cost trend crisis, they are a nonstarter. Look again at the people on the right-hand side of the cost continuum. One day in the hospital quickly blows past the $1,000 deductible and makes any cost-containment personal incentive features moot.

That's where the dollars are—not on the left with the already healthy. Any program that ignores the right-hand segment of the cost continuum is destined to fail.

Also, the mathematics can get quite complicated. If the people at the far left of the continuum who currently use no care at all select an MSA, they already cost nothing. So cutting their costs isn't possible. How can anyone use zero care so efficiently that they save the $500 or $1,000 in new cash that has been placed in their accounts by the MSAs?

Another somewhat ironic flaw in the typical MSA design is that the programs as currently designed and implemented have not actually, in any real sense, been "defined contribution." The whole point of defined contribution in the pension world for the employer is to limit the cost to the employer. An MSA, by contrast, has what is really unlimited top-end liability. Anyone who is sick enough to spend the entire deductible amount moves on to the insured portion of the benefit package. That insured portion tends to have unlimited coverage, with most employers self-insuring the full, unlimited benefits.

In other words, the MSA product is marketed as "defined contribution" without having the ultimate total contribution defined. That's clever marketing but not necessarily well-informed purchasing.

Street Market Vouchers

Another version of defined contribution that has been proposed by some benefit designers has been a pure voucher system in which employers would give each worker a voucher and let them go to the individual health insurance marketplace and buy coverage. Theorists claim that market model would open up competition in the insurance world and encourage workers to make wise insurance choices.

The problem with that theory is that it flies directly in the face of actuarial research and reality. The companies that sell individual insurance policies have no interest in enrolling sick people. Take another look at Figure 13.1. Insurers would love to enroll the people on the left side of the continuum. If the insurer can charge an average price and enroll those healthy people, the process would be very profitable for the insurer. Insurers who sell coverage in the individual market use careful underwriting practices to screen out the people on the right side of the continuum. Any insurance company in the country would go broke in a hurry if it charged an average premium and then enrolled the higher-cost 10 percent of the population.

The whole principle of insurance is that the premium from the houses that are not burning pay for the houses that are burning. If you insure only burning houses, the premium has to exceed the value of each house.

Giving workers vouchers and telling them to buy individual insurance would work for most of the healthy people but would result in no coverage at all for the unhealthy. That sort of defeats the whole concept of offering health insurance.

To make matters even more complicated, there's another cost chart that needs to be understood. Figure 13.2 shows total average annual health care costs by age. As you can see, people in their twenties have much lower average health care costs than people in their sixties.

Insurance companies that sell health insurance to individuals know these tables well and rate their products accordingly. A sixty year old who is buying coverage has to spend a lot more than a twenty year old who is buying the same benefit package. Why is that relevant to the voucher option? Because a voucher that works well for an average worker at age thirty buys great coverage for a twenty year old and pays only half the premium for a sixty year old. Age discrimination issues might surface at that point for employers.

Figure 13.2. Average U.S. Health Care Costs by Age

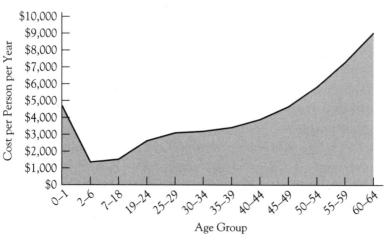

Source: Milliman USA Health Cost Guidelines—2001 Claim Probability Distributions.

In any case, some of the pure voucher advocates say that they are modeling their proposal after the 401(k) pension plans. Not true. Employers who offer 401(k) plans do not give their workers pension vouchers and tell them to go to the street market to make some kind of investment. 401(k) vouchers cannot be used for lottery tickets or penny stocks.

401(k) offerings are done in a carefully structured context with a limited number of carefully selected options, each vouched for as credible by a 401(k) administrator. The good 401(k) administrators offer a wide range of services to the workers, including information about the past performance of each investment option. Every worker is guaranteed a choice. They don't have to find a choice.

That model does not resemble the health care voucher proposal that calls for each employee to seek out his or her own benefit vendor and insurer.

401(k) Clones Might Work

An option that employers may find more useful is one that carefully emulates the 401(k) pension model. In the 401(k) clone, employers will hire an administrator to perform functions similar to the 401(k) pension administrator. In health care, that administrator will bring an array of benefit options to each employee group, along with data and information about each choice. The employer will offer a voucher, and each employee will have the opportunity to spend that voucher in the context of the benefit choices available.

Each benefit level and care system option will have a price. Richer benefits will be more expensive than skimpier benefits. Employees will be able to spend their voucher and add any additional cash from their own paycheck if they want to buy either the most comprehensive coverage or the least efficient care delivery approach. Proponents of that model say it moves away from the one-size-fits-all benefit approach with all key decisions made by the employer to a more flexible approach that lets employees make trade-offs between cost and value.

The obvious flaw in the model is that if it is set up poorly, it can lead to major levels of selection that will destroy the risk pool for any given group. If, for example, two carriers are offered side by side—one with a $1,000 deductible and a low price and the other with full coverage and a higher price—then the healthy people will migrate to the lower-benefit, low-price plan. The plan with the higher benefits will then need to raise its rates in an attempt to break even. Those rate increases, however, will backfire and cause even more people to find the lower-benefit/low-cost plan attractive. In just a couple of years, that cycle can make the high benefit plan unaffordable for all but the sickest patients. We've seen it happen.

That cycle ends with the viability of complete coverage being destroyed. Everyone is forced into lower benefits. Risk avoidance becomes the main agenda of the insurers. That's not a good outcome if one of the goals is to insure as many people as possible with adequate coverage.

What can be done about that situation? One way that Health-Partners dealt with that situation in Minnesota was to offer a wide array of benefit options through a single carrier. Us. Inside each risk pool, we arranged the pricing so that although there were meaningful price differences between the highest and lowest benefit levels, there also continued to be a cross subsidy from the people on the left side of the cost continuum to the people on the right. Without that cross subsidy, the more comprehensive benefit pool would have gone into what is generally referred to as an "actuarial death spiral."

Inside that melded risk pool, people were given choices; they could select a more tightly coordinated care network, or a loosely assembled non-network made up of totally independent providers. The non-network, of course, had both higher expense and lower scores on various areas of quality performance.

The Internet was used to provide information to consumers about those various choices and options and was also used for enrollments into each option. The employers didn't have to be involved in any of those processes. Just as employers now delegate those pension administration functions to a program administrator, employers in Minnesota were able to delegate their administrative tasks to the health plan 401(k) clone function.

Other carriers around the country are attempting to set up similar models. In some communities, buyer coalitions and benefit consultant houses are working to do something very similar.

In settings where multiple insurers and health plans are used, it will be critically important to make sure that there are clear and adequate risk-sharing and risk-adjustment formulas in place before enrollment even begins so that the carriers with the lower benefits will not simply be able to skim the best risks out of each risk pool.

The best 401(k) pension plan administrators offer a wide range of information-sharing approaches for their customers. With the best administrators, everyone can check the track record of each investment option and check on the daily status of each investment.

There's also a screening process. The administrators try to make sure that the investment options they offer are credible, viable, and ethical—if not profitable.

In the best of all worlds, similar value would be added for employee choices in a health care benefit option function. Ideally, the choices would not be simply actuarial, with benefit variations as the main differentiator. Ideally, consumers should have information about the quality of care as well as the extent of the benefits. Ideally, at least some of the choices ought to be focused on improving people's health, systematically improving the quality of care, and systematically improving both the efficiency and the accessibility of the care system.

A passive voucher-based marketplace that simply offers benefit choices can have a temporary impact on costs for an employer. An infrastructure that offers choices while actively improving care and patient health has a better chance of making a positive long-term difference for employers and employees.

Care improvement can be encouraged and rewarded if the choice marketplace features information about those functions. It will not be rewarded if those functions are not part of the process.

Experiments in Minnesota have shown that employees like choices and that those choices will gravitate toward higher-quality and more efficient care when those options are presented as part of the agenda.

Health care will not be focused on achieving either best practice or highest value unless both of those issues are recognized and rewarded. A carefully structured choice marketplace can create both that recognition and that reward. A badly designed marketplace will simply perpetuate the worst of today's nonsystem: paying lower benefits and creating some financial pain for selected patients but having no real impact on any of the factors that are increasing the cost of care.

14

Most Health Care Costs Are
the Result of Bad Health

It's a fairly basic point to make, but it's worth remembering that almost all health care costs are caused by health problems. Diseases create expense; preventing or avoiding diseases can reduce expenses. The very best disease prevention programs are, ultimately, both best care for patients and a best strategy for cost management.

This piece of information is particularly relevant in America today. We are increasingly obese and inert. We are more overweight as a nation than at any other time in our history. To make matters worse, we are also less physically active than at any other time in our history.

Now add to those factors the actuarial reality that we are also, on average, older than at any other time in our history. Anyone who understands the basic and direct relationships between weight, activity level, and age would be able to predict a major increase in our health care costs.

In an aging, inert, and obese population, chronic care diseases are a particular problem. The number of chronic care patients is increasing at an incredible rate. Chronic care treatment now uses over one-third of our total health care dollars. Within a couple of years, chronic care costs will exceed 80 percent of our total spending.[1] The number of people with diabetes in America, for example, has increased by one-third in a decade, and those numbers are growing, not shrinking.

The good news is that most of the complications of chronic diseases can be prevented or significantly delayed with aggressive and systematic health improvement campaigns targeted strategically at each disease. These programs, done well, have been proven to cut the complications of many chronic diseases by 50 percent or more. Some programs have even been able to help people avoid certain diseases entirely. That's why the third national strategic initiative proposed by this book is an aggressive population health improvement program.

We strongly recommend the use of systematic, outcomes-based care for the treatment of acute diseases to improve both the safety and outcomes of care. We are equally enthusiastic in our support for the application of systematic evidence-based approaches to preventing both acute and chronic disease.

Many Diseases Are Due to Behaviors

It's time for Americans to take a look at the impact that poor health is having on health care costs. Then we need to be honest with ourselves about causes of the chronic diseases that are absorbing our health care resources.

A number of diseases, such as some cancers or multiple sclerosis, have not been proven to result from the behavioral choices of patients. We also know, however, that major cost pressures in this country today do result from diseases that are, for the most part, consequences of unhealthy behaviors. Type II diabetes, for example, can be prevented, more often than not by appropriate behavior and diet changes. As noted earlier, we've seen a 33 percent increase in the number of people with diabetes in the United States since 1990. The reasons are diet and activity levels. We eat foods that make us vulnerable to diabetes and heart disease and then don't exercise enough to keep those diseases from taking over our bodies. A recent study found that the risk of diabetes was cut by 58 percent in patients who received counseling about weight loss, diet, and exercise.[2] Yet the health care nonsystem does a terrible job of helping us understand our risks or changing our behaviors.

Studies show that about half of all American adults and 11 percent of children are overweight. In the past twenty years, adult obesity has increased 50 percent.[3] And there are 4 to 10 million Americans whose physician considers them to be morbidly obese: 100 pounds or more overweight.[4]

Lack of physical activity, that is, a sedentary lifestyle, is one of the major underlying causes of death in this country. A 1996 surgeon general's report found that well over half of all Americans are physically inactive and that 25 percent are not active at all.[5] Physical activity may prevent or delay the onset of such diseases as diabetes, heart disease, stroke, gallbladder disease, some cancers, sleep apnea, high blood pressure, high cholesterol, and osteoarthritis.[6]

As physical fitness levels decrease, the likelihood of having one or more chronic conditions increases. A recent study showed significant excess medical expenses associated with low physical activity levels and fitness. Each additional day of physical activity per week per individual resulted in a 4.7 percent reduction of excess health care costs. For individuals in poor or fair fitness categories, there was an excess expense of $176 more per year than those who are moderately fit.[7] Those issues are particularly important for people who already have a chronic disease. The same study showed that the three-year costs of caring for people with diabetes ranged from $10,439 for those without heart disease and hypertension to $44,417 for those with those conditions. This study concluded that physical inactivity translates into significantly higher health care charges within a relatively short time period of eighteen months. The savings that could be realized simply by getting the sedentary to be more active are huge.

Health Disparities Among Different Ethnic and Racial Groups

To complicate matters further, we are also seeing wide disparities in health status by ethnicity and race. If we are going to improve the nation's health overall, we need to pay special attention to those populations with the most significant health problems.

When we see data comparing the United States to other industrialized countries, the numbers usually show the United States lagging behind in a number of key areas. We too often think of that as a general problem and wonder why our health is worse than that of the French or Germans even though we spend a lot more money on care. These numbers don't make any intuitive sense. They also aren't very useful in helping to set health policy because they don't point out the real opportunity for care improvement in the United States: our minority populations. Those numbers need to be more widely known.

According to the Office of Research on Minority Health (ORMH), African American, American Indians and Alaska Natives, Asian and Pacific Islander, and Hispanic citizens suffer significantly poorer health and higher rates of premature death than the majority population. Those groups also have higher rates of heart disease, lupus, diabetes, HIV/AIDS, end-stage renal disease, and certain cancers.[8] The following diseases or conditions strike at minority populations particularly hard.

Infant Mortality

Infant mortality in the United States has declined in the past few decades and in 1998 stood at a record low of 7.2 per 1,000 live births. However, the United States still ranks twenty-third in infant mortality among industrialized countries. Infant death rates among blacks, American Indians and Alaskan Natives, and Hispanics are all far above the national average. The greatest disparity exists for blacks, with an infant death rate of 13.9 per 1,000, over twice the rate for white infants (6.0 per 1,000).[9] Efforts to improve these rates must focus on modifying specific targeted behaviors such as smoking, substance abuse, and poor nutrition and on increasing prenatal care.[10]

Cancer

Cancer is the second leading cause of death in the United States, with more than 544,000 deaths each year. Many minority groups suffer disproportionately from cancer. African Americans have a cancer death rate that is 35 percent higher than·that for whites. The incidence of lung cancer is about 50 percent higher for black men than white men. Alaskan Natives have higher rates of colon and rectum cancer than whites. Vietnamese women in the United States have a cervical cancer incidence rate that is more than five times greater than that of white women (47.3 versus 8.7 per 100,000).

Evidence suggests that diet and nutrition may be related to 30 to 40 percent of cancers. Regular screening for breast cancer, colorectal cancer, and cervical cancer can help reduce the risk for these cancers, yet many minorities have low screening rates. These low rates may be due to limited access to health care or to barriers related to language or culture. In some cases, insensitive or negative provider attitudes may be a factor.[11]

We as a society have a need to recognize the challenging health impact of the major recent waves of immigration. Tens of millions of new Americans from Africa, Asia, and South America bring whole new ranges of health care problems to the American health scene. Most U.S. doctors aren't prepared to deal with the parasites and diseases of less developed countries, but many doctors are now forced to deal with them regularly.

Cardiovascular Disease

Cardiovascular disease and stroke kill nearly as many Americans as all other diseases combined in the United States. The annual economic impact of cardiovascular disease is estimated at $259 billion. Again, major disparities exist among population groups. Racial and ethnic minorities have higher rates of hypertension and are less likely to undergo treatment to control their high blood pressure. The age-adjusted death rate for heart disease for the total population declined by 20 percent from 1987 to 1995; for blacks, the overall decline was only 13 percent. Regular screening for cholesterol also varies greatly by ethnic groups. In 1997, 67 percent of African Americans, 59 percent of Hispanics, 68 percent of Asians, and 55 percent of American Indians and Alaskan Natives had their cholesterol checked within the past five years as compared to 71 percent of whites.[12]

Diabetes

Diabetes now affects nearly 16 million Americans. The prevalence of diabetes in blacks is about 70 percent higher than it is for whites. For Hispanics, the prevalence is nearly double that of whites. Among American Indians and Alaskan Natives, the rate is more than twice that for the total population, and at least one tribe, the Pimas in Arizona, have the world's highest prevalence rate of diabetes. (Interestingly, across the border in adjacent Mexico, members of the same Pima tribe eat different food, exercise more, and are only one-third as likely to suffer from the disease.)

Cardiovascular disease is the leading cause of death among people with diabetes. Preventive efforts to reduce mortality from diabetes will require targeted efforts to reduce cardiovascular risk factors. This is particularly challenging since for every two people who are aware of their diabetes, one person remains undiagnosed.[13] More often than not, the undiagnosed person is a member of a minority group.

HIV/AIDS

HIV/AIDS is now the leading cause of death for persons twenty-five to forty-four years of age. AIDS also disproportionately affects minority populations. Roughly 25 percent of the entire U.S. population is made up of racial and ethnic minorities, yet the minority citizens account for nearly 54 percent of all AIDS cases. AIDS death rates actually declined by 23 percent for the total U.S. population during the mid-1990s but declined only 13 percent for African Americans and 20 percent for Hispanics. Inadequate recognition of risk, detection of infection, and referral to follow-up care are major issues for minority populations.[14]

AIDS is yet another disease for which medical science can now provide miracles. People with AIDS now live for many years, thanks primarily to new drugs and treatments. The drugs are costly, however, so the cost implications of keeping AIDS patients alive are very similar to the situation of kidney dialysis patients discussed in Chapter One.

Until There Is a National Plan, Implement Local Plans

Clearly, the United States needs a national health policy aimed at improving population health in a number of key areas. As we set our goals, we need to place a particular emphasis on making sure we are focusing enough energy and resources on the minority populations with the highest level of health problems.

We need to be insightful in not attributing all differences in disease patterns to societal issues. In doing that, we can overlook genetic issues that need to be specifically addressed. A genetic susceptibility to diabetes, for example, should not be ignored; it should be the foundation for aggressive treatment, education, and prevention agendas. (One of us has ancestors who were Native American. Just about every member of the family on that side becomes diabetic in their fifties or sixties. That ought to be preventable— but only if the genetic susceptibility is known and then taken into consideration.)

Until we can put together a comprehensive national strategy, however, we should do what we can with health plan–specific disease prevention programs. There's no point in waiting until the government acts. Based on experience, that could be a while. Currently, the nation has established some goals: the Healthy People 2010 goals created by the U.S. Department of Health and Human Services.[15] They are a positive first step, but as a nation, we have not committed resources or created programs to reach those goals. We have goals but no strategies to achieve them. Until the government decides to act, we ought to make use of the best tools at hand for improving population health: health plans. We believe that health plans can have a huge positive impact on the health of their members now if the plans are committed to a population health agenda and if the plans work in close partnership with their provider networks and patients.

Guidelines for a Prevention Agenda and Health Program

What should a prevention agenda and population health program look like for a health plan? That's a question we've wrestled with for the better part of a decade. Over that time, we've come to some conclusions about how health plans and their medical group partners can most effectively improve population health.

Plans Should Set Quantifiable Health Improvement Goals

Plans and their medical group partners should start by setting goals, measurable goals, to be met in a defined period of time. We believe that any prevention-focused plan health program that doesn't start with concrete goals will not know where to put its energy or how to assign its resources most effectively. A program without goals too often pays lip-service to prevention but fails to take the steps necessary to actually prevent anything.

It's clear that local health plans can both set population health goals and achieve them. Health plans and their provider partners can cut the number of people who become diabetic and the number of people who have heart attacks. In the best of all worlds, sophisticated buyers should insist on selecting or favoring plans that set those goals and then implement real programs to achieve them.

What should a health plan goal look like? Here are some examples from Minnesota:

- Reduce the rate of congestive heart failure hospitalizations by 50 percent.

- Reduce the incidence of suicide attempts and suicide among depressed members by 50 percent.

- Reduce the number of high-risk patients who become diabetic by 25 percent.

- Reduce tobacco use among adults from 25 percent to 15 percent.

These goals are measurable, they are possible, and they can be accomplished. They are inspirational to the point that they inspire creative thinking among the caregivers whose support is essential to the achievement of each goal.

Each of those goals gives strategic direction to a plan. We know that they provide useful direction, because they are all among the goals we've already set for the Partners for Better Health 2005 Program at HealthPartners in Minnesota. Each represents major movement—and major improvements—over prior levels of care. We know from experience that when the brightest and best caregivers in a health plan or medical group get together to figure out how to turn these goals into reality, the goals inspire creative thinkers to figure out ways of making better health very real.

A plan that decides to cut second heart attacks by 25 percent starts by measuring current performance levels. Then the caregivers figure out what approaches to care and patient education can achieve these goals. Aspirin distribution becomes a crusade, not just an afterthought. Beta blocker distribution becomes an urgent mission.

HealthPartners achieved a 98 percent success level on beta blockers in Minnesota; the national average is roughly half that number. (The national number is a crime.) As noted earlier, beta blockers cut second heart attacks by roughly 40 percent. Our health plan's huge beta blocker success would not have happened without a systematic prevention program aimed at achieving a clearly defined goal.

In northern California, the Kaiser Permanente program for reducing both heart disease and heart attacks has been so successful that heart disease has fallen to be the second leading cause of death among Kaiser Permanente members, although heart disease remains the number one cause of death in the general population. Systematic approaches to care do work to improve health.

How does a plan, medical group, or care system set up a systematic prevention program? HealthPartners started in Minnesota by using a health improvement model as the foundation for planning for each priority condition. This model, shown in Figure 14.1, is referred to informally as the bubble chart, or sometimes, "Isham's Bubbles," in honor of George Isham who invented and first used it.

For each targeted disease (for example, diabetes, asthma, heart disease, depression), we figure out who in our current population is in which category of care. For those people in the far-right bubble—people with active disease—we provide best care. We use best care protocols to move people out of that bubble, back to the left.

Figure 14.1. HealthPartners Health Improvement Model

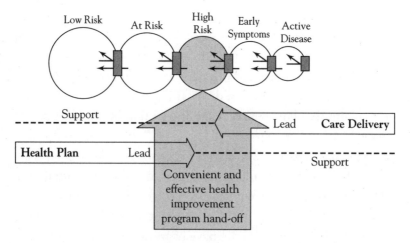

Source: Copyright © HealthPartners 2002. Partners for Better Health 2005.

Focus First on the People at Risk

For people in the at-risk or high-risk categories, we put specific programs in place to change behavior and reduce risk. Beta blockers and aspirin are used for patients at high risk of heart attacks. HealthPartners tailors programs and approaches to help high-risk people lower their risk for each disease.

For the people on the far left of Figure 14.1, in the low-risk bubble, we do relatively little. We do provide some health information, but those people are not our best opportunities to change lives. It's a waste of time, money, and energy to preach excessively to the converted.

Far too many programs that purport to be prevention programs actually focus most of their energy on the population in that bubble on the far left. In too many programs, healthy people are encouraged to join health clubs. Nonsmokers are urged to continue not to smoke.

Those efforts mean well, but they are part of the reason that too many employers now don't support health agendas for their employees. When the healthy are simply urged to stay that way and the less healthy people don't get special attention, any positive payback for the employer is a long time in coming.

By contrast, when the focus is on people at risk, the payback can be almost immediate. Asthma is a good example. If a system identifies all asthma patients, makes sure every asthma patient gets the right drugs and care, and then invites all patients into group counseling programs to learn to avoid and manage asthma crisis, the financial payback for the employer happens overnight. Hospital admissions for asthma crisis drop in half quickly. People lead much healthier lives very quickly. Better health means lower premiums and a more valuable workforce because people are on the job instead of at home recovering from an asthma crisis.

Buyers and policymakers need to realize that the science of prevention has improved dramatically in recent years. Targeted intervention now makes a real difference in improving and maintaining people's health. Care improves. Savings result.

Buyers Must Demand Actual Health Improvement Goals

The best incentive for plan health improvement programs is buyer demand. Buyers of health coverage must ask plans for their actual health improvement objectives. Bouquets of four-color brochures or a high-sounding recitation of health rhetoric are not enough. Buyers should ask each plan for a list of concrete prevention goals. They should ask what specific things are being done by the plan and its providers to achieve these goals. They should ask exactly which people they are being done for. They should seek evidence that the plan's health objectives are actually being achieved and request materials being used with real patients to achieve these goals. And they ought to talk to the caregivers who are directly improving health for individual patients.

If these questions can't be answered, then the plan has a marketing campaign, not a health improvement program.

Disease prevention is too important and far too valuable to be left solely to the advertising and public relations departments. The potential gain of a healthy on-the-job workforce is too important not to be a conscious part of a buyer's purchasing criteria. Buyers will get only what they insist on buying. Until the government creates a cohesive prevention program, buyers must insist that health plans accomplish that goal. It can be done.

National Strategy, Plan-Level Implementation

This chapter calls for a long-term national health improvement strategy and a short-term local health plan strategy. We believe the government should support programs that cut congestive heart failure crisis, asthma crisis, and flu deaths by more than half. That support can take several forms: government funds for research into how to prevent diseases; insistence on preventive care as a benefit for government program beneficiaries; and laws, where needed, to allow for programs and data use that facilitate population-based care improvement.

Buyers can, and should, go a step further and reward the best care systems now for doing a good job on improving population health. Buyer rhetoric won't get the job done on its own. Buyer rhetoric combined with buyer behavior adequately reinforced with buyer dollars could very quickly transform the marketplace for the better and improve the health of all Americans.

Prevention can create real value for everyone concerned.

15

. . . .

Caregiver Monopolies Should Not
Be Our Care Model of Choice

The fourth major policy initiative deals with keeping the health care marketplace competitive. Market forces will never affect health care costs positively if state and federal lawmakers allow caregivers to form local monopolies and oligopolies.

This shouldn't be a surprise to anyone who understands economic forces. Monopolies in any industry tend to inflate prices and profits at the expense of the buyer. Health care is no exception. The difference is, however, that monopolies in health care can be very local, whereas monopolies in other industries tend to be much larger and therefore much more visible.

In health care, we've already seen new monopolies and oligopolies jack up prices from 10 to 200 percent over the past couple of years. These cost increases are having a direct, immediate, and permanent impact on consumer premiums. The likelihood of a rollback on those prices is almost nil, at least as the health care delivery market is constructed today.

Higher prices, however, are not the most frustrating problem that results from provider monopolies. Lower-quality care is. Uncompetitive markets in health care work against consumers' best interests and likelihood of receiving best care because providers that control markets have little or no incentive to improve either service or care in order to remain competitive. Health care is no different from any other area of the economy. It's pretty hard to persuade people to work extra hard to improve service levels when everyone on the scene knows that there will be just as many customers (or patients) if both service and care are mediocre, or even bad.

Noncompetitive providers can wallow safely in the local status quo. Persuading innovative caregivers to integrate care around the patient works best when the clear alternative is to lose the patient to a high-performing competitor. The changes needed at the next level in health care are all challenging. Care coordination is wonderful, but it's hard to do and takes a lot of work. It requires boundary blurring in multiple care settings. People hate to have their boundaries blurred. Persuading a complacent, monopolistic caregiver staff to restructure systems and reengineer approaches around patient convenience is almost impossible when there's no obvious and compelling competitive advantage that will result from the restructuring.

Systematic improvement of service and care can, we know, be done in an extremely well-led monopolistic organization with an exceptional internal commitment to excellence. There are a few examples we could point to where that has happened, but such organizations are few and far between.

A standard rule of monopolies in any setting is that the convenience priorities of all participants revolve around the interests of the monopolist, not the customer.

If Uncompetitive Markets Exist, Demand Performance Data

It's far too easy for caregivers to create monopolies in most areas of the country. As noted in Chapter Five, caregiver monopolies don't have to cover very large geographical areas to jack up prices because market realities have shown pretty clearly that patients will not drive very far for their care. Monopolies in health care can and do happen at a very local level. In some areas, due to low local population levels, uncompetitive markets are formed automatically by the fact that there aren't enough patients to support two caregivers. In those settings, we believe some levels of competitive pressure can still apply. That competitive pressure can come from data. Buyers and health plans can collect data and report them to the public. What good are data in noncompetitive settings? The information sets up benchmarks and expectations, and it makes people smarter about the value of their care.

In areas where local care monopolies already exist, buyers and consumers would benefit from public information about the relative costs and care performance levels of the local caregivers. Those data can be compared to equivalent data from other locations.

Even if the local market has no competition, important pieces of information about prices and care outcomes in those consolidated areas could still be compared with comparable information from other unconsolidated markets.

Local consumers should at least be aware that a local hospital stay costs 25 to 50 percent more than an equivalent stay in a competitive market, for example. Or that local beta blocker compliance is only at 47 percent, compared to a statewide level of 60 percent or a local health plan average of 98 percent.

That information would let the community become both informed and more knowledgeable purchasers of care. It would also allow the community to help the local care system target areas for improvement. Without that information, local improvement plans are unlikely to happen. With it, community support for targeted care improvement can benefit all parties. Only data allow the creation of those targets.

The exact mechanism for getting that performance information into public view can vary. Aggregated payer data could do the job in some settings. If all local payments are done on a fee basis, simple public reports showing comparative fee schedules and unit prices would be a good start. That data could be gathered by a third party from all payers and then melded to show the people in each community, on average, what they are paying for care.

Local caregivers could be required to produce those data about their own performance as a legal consequence of being allowed to form a local monopoly. State and federal attorneys are sometimes involved in approving or disapproving the formation of local monopolies. When our regulators approve the new monopolies, they should minimally require extensive ongoing performance reporting as a condition of the deal.

A lot of performance promises are typically made to the public in advance of large provider mergers. The silence on those same topics is deafening once the merger has been consolidated. At most, negotiators take a generic look at the merger aftermath in some form of highly choreographed hearings a few years later. The hearings tend to be much less useful than a publication of public comparative fee, cost, and outcome reporting imposed on the caregivers at the time of mergers. Like many courtship situations, the very best promises are often extracted prior to the consortium. Let's make that fact work for the public.

Having information about prices and care quality will let consumers know when local problems exist relative to important areas of care. Even if there are no local competitors for patients to move to, the mere knowledge of problem areas can help citizens direct some level of community moral suasion at local provider pricing decisions or care levels.

In communities where moral suasion doesn't work, at least local people will know exactly why their local health insurance premiums are so high.

In other instances, those data will give local consumers the peace of mind that comes from knowing that local provider prices are fair and local care meets or exceeds reasonable standards.

In either instance, comparative data enable local consumers and caregivers to start a community dialogue about care system needs and performance that probably will not otherwise happen.

Regulators Need to Wake Up

In areas of the country where provider consolidation hasn't yet reached critical mass, antitrust people need to be more active. The standards of competition applied to health care up to this point have not been sufficient to protect the public interest. Regulators need a much more sophisticated understanding of how health care markets actually work.

It's futile to attempt to introduce competition into every health care marketplace. It's good public policy, however, to support, rein-force, and protect competition in those markets where it now exists. Both antitrust regulators and purchasers of health care services should have as a goal the protection of competition in most markets.

Time is of the essence. This is an area that shouldn't be left to chance. We don't have time to do extensive, long-term studies of the issues because the consolidation is already going on. A national study just done by the University of Minnesota pointed out that horizontal mergers within provider specialties are occurring now in many major markets.[1] Hospital merger trends are also prevalent in most markets.

Antitrust laws need to be invoked at a very local level, or provider competition will disappear in key areas in hundreds of markets.

What About Health Plan Mergers?

Competition is the best force for improving health care quality and containing prices. Just as consumers are hurt by provider monopolies, so too can they be hurt by total market dominance by any single health plan. What about the danger of health plan mergers? Don't those mergers also drive up premiums?

Any mergers will drive up premiums if the result is a functional monopoly.

Antitrust people also need to be very careful not to allow any given health plan to take over a market. Actual levels of meaningful competition for insurance products can exist with only two or three plans in any given market, but, with few exceptions, single-plan markets will not provide local citizens or buyers with the benefits of competition unless the prices of the plans in those markets mirror the prices and margins of those plans in fully competitive markets.

However, some degree of market consolidation by local health plans may be strategically needed if local providers merge. One major value provided to consumers by health plans is to use volume leverage to reduce provider fees. As providers get to be huge, the balance of negotiating power shifts to higher fees. In those settings, plans may also need to get larger. The economic logic is pretty basic. Plans with small market share often have a very hard time getting solid discounts from large, market-dominant providers of care. Without these discounts, plan premiums can be significantly more expensive. Consumers, of course, suffer. When providers get big, plans must also grow in order to negotiate good prices for their members.

Some policymakers and economists, not understanding the real-world dynamics of health care purchasing, have stated that "ten or more" health plans are needed to keep any given insurance market competitive. The people making those statements have obviously never been face to face with a provider over a negotiating table. That perspective might have been true at one time when providers were a lot smaller and had less leverage. In highly consolidated provider markets, however, they are wrong, even dangerously wrong. Markets with ten or more plans would be a consolidated megacaregiver's dream. In that market, no health plan would ever have any real negotiating leverage.

To the contrary, if a market had consolidated providers and ten equally sized health plans, all ten plans would be at the pricing mercy of the consolidated providers, particularly if the providers have already merged into zip code monopolies. In a ten-plan market, any zip code–dominant provider could raise prices easily by simply threatening any given plan with leaving it if the provider's price demands weren't met.

If two or three plans hold most of the market, those plans can still each negotiate good deals with even large caregivers. But if a market has ten or more small plans that share the market equally, the big provider wins. Although the economic logic is fairly simple, many policymakers have yet to grasp it.

Why does that particular negotiating situation suddenly give providers more leverage than plans? This is an important point that few policymakers understand. It's really very simple. Look at the relative consequences to each party of a "failed" negotiation. If a market has ten or more health plans of roughly equal size, then any provider group that decides to hold up any single plan for higher costs would lose 10 percent of its patients at worst. That would happen only if the plan got tough, executed its bluffs, and stopped using the provider. That loss would be painful to the provider but not crippling. Most providers can handle a loss of 10 percent of their patients, particularly if the trade-off is a 15 percent increase in revenue from the remaining 90 percent of the patients. More money, less work.

Also, in many cases, the real patient loss number for the provider with a cancelled health plan contract would be somewhat lower than 10 percent, because many of the canceled plan's patients would simply switch health plans and return at open enrollment to that same provider with a different plan's ID card in their wallet. Most providers contract with multiple plans.

By contrast, a health plan suddenly faced with a major hole in its geographical distribution would stand to lose much more, possibly becoming highly noncompetitive for some buyers in comparison to other local health plans that don't have that same hole in their provider network. The plan itself might no longer be a viable option for many buyers. We've seen plans with large geographical voids lose well over 10 percent of their membership in a year. And that particular plan would find itself in an even weaker position when the next locally dominant caregiver makes that same plan another high price demand.

What does the plan do then?

A network with two major holes is even more crippled in the marketplace than a network with one hole. So the price increases from the second round are often accepted, and plan costs go up accordingly.

When the consequences to each party in a negotiation are that vastly uneven, who wins? That's easy. Who loses? The real losers are consumers, who have to pay a lot more for their premiums and their care.

When Buyers Offer Only One Plan, Provider Leverage Increases

Ironically, in some markets, buyer behavior sets the stage for provider price increases. In the early days of HMOs, most employers offered multiple health plans to the employees. Over time, the number of plans offered by any given employer has been shrinking, and some employers now offer only one or two plans. That seemingly innocuous change in purchasing behavior has had a major unintended impact on the balance of power in plan-provider negotiations.

Why?

In a marketplace where employers offered multiple plans, no single plan had to have complete geographical coverage. If one plan didn't offer providers on the south side of town, for example, another plan would probably have those providers. In aggregate, all plans would have covered all geography. Since even very small employers typically have employees who live in sites scattered all over the local geographical area, plan network coverage of the entire area is usually seen as a necessity for the buyer. Multiple plans met that need easily. No single plan needed to be everywhere, because one plan void was another plan network.

When most employers cut back to offering only one or two plans, however, the situation changed. In those circumstances, each plan must cover the entire geographical area. Plans with partial geographical coverage tend to lose business. At this time, as one major hospital system CEO says very succinctly, "Geography is power." When each employer offers only one or two plans, the negotiating leverage of geography-dominant local providers goes up, way up, and prices go up accordingly.

Clearly, a balance needs to be struck for both providers and plans. Policymakers and attorneys general need to be aware of the dangers of monopolies relative to pricing, service levels, and the quality of care.

For much of the country, that horse is already out of the barn. In many major communities, the time for damage prevention is gone; only damage control is still a possibility.

Purchasers Should Be Able to Trigger Antitrust Reform

If we are going to set up a national health initiative to foster competition on that issue, we ought to require the antitrust regulators to look rigorously into any proposed provider merger in any market that gives majority market share to any caregiver or set of caregivers. That scrutiny should extend to all types of specialists, as well as to hospitals and the more obvious larger providers.

Any purchaser should be able to trigger antitrust review of caregivers when that level of consolidation is threatened. Likewise, any provider should be able to trigger formal antitrust review of any insurer or health plan merger when the result will be a monopoly marketplace.

In cases where mergers are allowed, the regulators should follow and study the price levels set by the newly merged entity for at least the next five years and should require the merged entity to do ongoing public reporting of both pricing and care performance levels.

A worst-case scenario would be to have each market in the United States owned by separate, dominant, monopoly caregivers in each area of care. That would be a marketplace of poor service, poor care coordination, and excessive prices. If we let that happen, we have only ourselves to blame. Anyone could see it coming.

16

· ·

Cut the Number of
Uninsured in Half

It is both sad and discouraging that America can spend $4,930 per citizen on health care and still have over 41.2 million Americans uninsured. As noted in Chapter Ten, the British provide universal health care coverage for every citizen of that country and do it for only $1,763 per Briton in tax dollars. We spend significantly more than that in tax dollars alone and three times that much overall, and we still leave far too many people with no coverage at all.

People who are uninsured tend to receive less care. Children who are uninsured receive a lot less care and often miss out entirely on the immunizations and well-baby checkups that are so important relative to the health and safety levels for each child.

People who are uninsured tend to wait longer before going to the doctor when they are sick. Letting cancer, heart disease, diabetes, or other diseases progress to bad points before seeking treatment can be a major health care mistake. Late treatment makes those conditions much harder to treat and decreases the likelihood of a cure or positive outcome. Uninsured people in America still get care, but they often get that care too late. At that point, health care bills can easily destroy a patient's personal financial status.

When people do delay care, the resultant bills can be unafford-able for most uninsured Americans. Then, when care has thoroughly impoverished the patient and family, the patient finally qualifies for Medicaid, and the government begins to pay for the rest of the treatment. In the process, people's lives and economic stability can be damaged, even destroyed.

It is particularly unfortunate that such a large portion of our uninsured are children. Our senior population has Medicare as a form of uninsured coverage for older Americans. All seniors are already covered by a single-payer system of sorts. By contrast, millions of our youngest citizens have no coverage at all.[1] These children often miss out entirely on the primary care services that are so important for the protection of their health and their ability to function well in school.

Interestingly, we already have programs in place that should be correcting a large portion of that problem for our children. Over half of America's uninsured children are already fully eligible for Medicaid or other subsidized care plans.[2] Those children could have free or very low-cost coverage if their parents knew about the program and simply filled in the proper forms. That's easier said than done, however. Those forms are a mess—a real challenge to complete. Because the bureaucratic barriers to their enrollment are too great for many parents, particularly single parents in high-stress situations, many eligible children do not receive Medicaid benefits. Part of the problem results from the fact that many low-income parents do not understand that their children are eligible. We don't seem to have good ways of getting that message to those parents in a useful and persuasive way. That could be fixed if we set our mind to it. Schools, clinics, and other settings could be used more effectively than they are today.

A large portion of the problem of uninsured children could be largely fixed under current programs by having the government create easier enrollment forms and procedures and then running more aggressive, persuasive, and effective education, outreach, and enrollment assistance programs for low-income parents.

We Already Pay for Most People's Care; We Just Make Them Broke First

Keep in mind that ultimately everyone in America is eligible for care once they are really sick. Each of us may not be eligible for "coverage," but everyone in the United States is eligible for care. Patients with dire conditions cannot legally be turned away from any hospital emergency rooms, even if they are impoverished and have absolutely no coverage. By law, hospitals must examine and treat them for serious medical conditions until they can be safely released.[3] A great many uninsured people know this now and use ERs for what is often basic care. The cost of caring for those uninsured patients is simply added to the bills of all insured patients as part of hospital overhead expenses. But using the emergency care system as the primary source of care for most of these patients is an incredibly inefficient, inconvenient, inappropriate, poorly timed, and wastefully expensive use of care resources. The poor patients who use the ER for their routine sicknesses as a care site of last resort would almost always have been better off seeing a doctor in a clinic, and the clinic visits would cost a lot less money.

When you consider the cost shifts from bad debt, combined with the mandatory hospital care provided to the truly ill, one can argue that the overall costs of care in this country already include much of the impact of caring for the uninsured. We just make the uninsured go through inconvenience and even misery to get that care, and then we pay for it in dysfunctional, indirect, inefficient, and unfair ways.

We clearly need a better system for taking care of uninsured Americans. In order to create that system, we first need to ask ourselves, Who exactly are the uninsured?

Who Are the Uninsured?

The answer to that question is slightly more complex than most people realize. There are actually several major categories of uninsured people: (1) people who are healthy or wealthy and don't feel a need to be insured, (2) people in transition between jobs or in transition between education and employment, (3) people who can't afford coverage, (4) people who have been rejected for health coverage because of their personal health status, and (5) employed people whose employers do not offer coverage. Of the 41.2 million uninsured, roughly 3 percent fall into category 1, 15 percent fall into category 2, 47 percent fall into category 3, 5 percent fall into category 4, and 15 percent fall into category 5.[4]

Each Category of Uninsured Needs Its Own Solution

Clearly, the solutions that will work for category 1 are not the same solutions needed for category 2, or 3, or 4, or 5. Each set of uninsured people has its own reason for being uninsured, and each group needs its own strategy to become insured.

Some categories of the uninsured obviously are in worse shape than others, so although our ultimate goal ought to be coverage of everyone, we should probably focus our immediate energy on those who are most in need of help.

If we are prioritizing our efforts, we probably don't need to do very much to help the people in transition. Typically, they are uninsured for twelve months or less. Many actually have access to some form of coverage and simply don't use it. People who have just left employment, for example, have clearly defined extended coverage rights under the COBRA laws. Individuals have sixty days after a "qualifying event" or after the employer has informed them of their eligibility to elect COBRA coverage.[5] They can continue that coverage for up to eighteen months. Those laws have an important and useful provision that allows people who have left a job to retroactively activate their group insurance coverage for up to eighteen months by paying a set premium.[6] Those premiums tend to be quite high, so most unemployed people don't pay them—until and unless they need them. Healthy but nonworking people seldom spend the necessary $800 or $1,000 a month to buy COBRA coverage.

So who usually buys COBRA extension coverage? The sick: people with cancer or heart disease, people who need surgery. If an unemployed person becomes really sick during that COBRA eligibility extension period, then the high premiums are a financial bargain. Sick people whose care expenses exceed the premiums tend to pay those premiums. They are then covered.

In effect, relative to any catastrophic care expenses clearly at hand, many people in transition between jobs are really not completely uninsured during that extension period. They simply haven't activated their insurance because they don't actually need it. Many people in transition would be better off with coverage, particularly people with families and a health problem of one kind or another. But most are healthy and relatively less likely to need care. This is not our highest priority need for coverage.

The Healthy and the Wealthy Uninsured Don't Need Much Help

The healthy and the wealthy uninsured also don't present a major issue. The young and healthy who choose not to buy coverage are, more often than not, people whose asset base and income levels are low enough to allow them to qualify fairly quickly for Medicaid if any real health problems emerge. Most young adults who are uninsured also tend to be low-risk people. They usually don't need a lot of care. Their health care costs are not our most pressing social issue.

The well-to-do uninsured can simply use their wealth to pay for any care they might need. Insurance for them isn't an issue. There's not much point in creating public programs designed to help the uninsured wealthy buy insurance.

If we want to move this country to full coverage, we could do that for both the healthy and the wealthy by simply requiring everyone to buy at least catastrophic coverage—perhaps coverage with a $5,000 deductible. That would cover the motorcycle accident that creates a brain-dead patient that costs some hospital $500,000 a year in bad debt or the wealthy stroke victim whose family may or may not be able to generate the cash flow needed for $100,000 in emergency care and subsequent rehabilitation. The premium for a high-deductible catastrophic plan for those people would be relatively cheap. We could use the tax system to collect those premiums annually from anyone who can't or won't show evidence of coverage when filing taxes. The healthy and the wealthy are not our highest-priority populations, however, so that solution could wait until the other problems of the truly sick and needy uninsured are resolved.

What About the People Rejected by Insurers?

The people who have attempted to buy coverage and whom insurers rejected are also a relatively small number. They are, however, a much higher-priority problem than the healthy and the wealthy because they need help. Unfortunately, by definition, these people all actually do have very real health care problems and needs, or the various private insurers would not have rejected them for coverage.

How can we provide coverage to these people? Again, the good news is that there is already an answer in place for most of them. According to the Agency for Health Care Policy and Research, thirty-one of fifty states have high-risk pools. The premiums, though subsidized, are not generally affordable for most people. These programs are typically somewhat underfunded, but they can be extremely useful in helping otherwise uninsurable people get coverage. These programs need to be extended in every state and funded from reasonable tax sources. Those programs fix most of the problem of the otherwise uninsurable fairly easily. The only issue is the cost.

In Minnesota, creating a program of that type increased the premiums paid by all insured Minnesotans by less than 2 percent.[7] Premiums paid by other people are used to subsidize coverage for the uninsured.

That Leaves the Working Uninsured

After the healthy and the wealthy uninsured, the uninsured in transition, and the uninsured who have been rejected by insurers, that leaves 62 percent of the uninsured working Americans whose employers don't offer coverage or feel that it is too expensive to purchase coverage through their employer. Most workers reject coverage because they have coverage elsewhere. However, a significant portion rejects coverage because they can't afford the employee share of premium.[8] In those cases, the employers usually make some contribution to the cost of coverage, but the remaining out-of-pocket expense for the employee is still too high.

One option for these people might be to leave the group market and buy individual coverage from an insurer. That approach sounds good, but it is not. Buying coverage in today's standard nongroup insurance market is truly not a good answer for most workers. Nongroup insurance coverage tends to be extremely expensive, in part because this insurance is inherently burdened with a huge administrative cost that group coverage does not have. The administrative cost is so high for very practical reasons: it costs a lot more per customer to sell and set up individual insurance coverage contracts than group contracts. Group coverage sold by an HMO typically has an administrative cost ranging from 6 to 15 percent. By contrast, individual insurance policies sold by an independent insurance agent typically have administrative cost burdens that range anywhere from 20 to 50 percent. That's a heavy load for a low-income worker to carry on top of the needed costs of care. In other words, 50 percent of the premium for individually sold insurance contracts can go to administrative overhead, and that doesn't count the portion of the premium needed for insurer profit.

Don't be too critical of the private insurers that offer those poli-cies. Surprisingly, that is not a conspiracy on their part to waste or steal people's money. Those administrative costs are, for the most part, real. It's very expensive to sell, service, and renew individual health insurance contracts.

It Costs a Lot Less to Bill One Hundred People at a Time

It's worth understanding those issues relative to evaluating the op-tions we have for dealing with the uninsured. Think about how the nongroup market works. Instead of sending out one bill for, say, one hundred covered lives (in an employer group setting), an insurer that sells coverage directly to individual people has to send out one hundred separate bills, one to each insured person or family. For starters, that's ninety-nine more stamps, ninety-nine more en-velopes. Then the insurer has to reconcile each bill against actual payments by each individual. That means ninety-nine more recon-ciliations. Every month, bad debt is much higher in the individual sales area as well.

The likelihood that a group bill to an employer for one hun-dred people might involve a bad check or lost paperwork is small. Employers tend to pay in full and pay on time. By contrast, the likelihood of having at least a few of the one hundred individual bills not being paid promptly or correctly in any given month is pretty high. But late payments do arrive, so coverage can't just be canceled at that point. Reinstatements happen all the time. Each takes the time of a billing clerk, who has to set up the late bills, re-build the computer file, and then recall and repay any claims that might have been suspended or rejected while it appeared that an individual member had cancelled coverage. That's a very expensive set of tasks. They happen over and over again in the individual di-rect sales marketplace.

Overall, it's a real headache, an expensive headache, to administer individual insurance contracts. It's a complex, labor-intensive process.

Those are just the internal administrative costs.

Sales Costs Are Also Heavy

Sales costs for individual contracts are equally disproportional relative to group coverage. Remember how the sales process for individual insurance works. People need to be persuaded to buy that coverage. It can take just about as much time, and sometimes longer, for an insurance agent to sell one individual policy as it does to sell a twenty-person group policy. People don't rush into decisions when they have to pay a big premium directly out of their own pocket.

Sales take time. If sales agents are paid by the hour, then the costs per covered life mount up hourly. If they are paid by commission, then the commission for an individual sale has to be a much larger percentage of the premium than a group sale or the agent can't afford to spend time selling to individuals.

A group sale commission charged by an agent might be only 1 percent of total premium or less. One percent of a $20,000 monthly premium for a small employer group is $200. What percentage of a $500 monthly premium is needed to make that sale worthwhile for an independent agent? Ten percent is only $50. Is that enough? An individual sale commission might need to be 10 percent to 20 percent or even more before it's worth an agent's time to attempt to make a direct sale, particularly since all insurers screen individual applicants for coverage. The agent has to help gather the health data and then will discover that some portion of the sales he or she made will be rejected by the underwriting staff of the health insurer or health plan.

Since not every prospect actually buys coverage, the agents need to be adequately compensated for the sales they do make.

It's possible that the Internet can be used to handle many of those marketing expenses to lower the distributed cost of the product. Even if that happens (and it is being done now in some settings), the administrative setup time for each member will still be more costly than group coverage.

What does all of that tell us? It says that expecting uninsured low-income people to buy coverage on the individual insurance market is generally not a good use of citizens' money. The people who end up paying those excess nongroup administrative costs are often those who can least afford it. Also, because individual coverage invariably is priced based on the age and sex of the insured person, that coverage can be highly unaffordable for any citizens over the age of forty. A sixty year old could easily be required to pay a thousand dollars a month or more for full family coverage. That isn't affordable for most people. It's a particular burden if the older person is semiretired. It takes a good part-time job to be able to pay a $1,000 per month premium from the after-tax proceeds.

Tax Credits Have Been Proposed

Some people have recommended the use of tax credits to fund coverage for this segment of the uninsured. The government would, in effect, subsidize the purchase of coverage by allowing for a reduction in taxes paid by the individual. People could buy individual coverage and then write off the cost of that coverage against their next year's taxes. Some tax credit advocates favor a plan that would create the equivalent of prospective vouchers to allow for an ongoing cost, often to subsidize immediate purchase of insurance. Policy experts who favor a nongovernment model often advocate the tax credit approach.

The approach might work well for some people, but many others would find that because the insurance market sets premiums based on age or health status and would still have a very high administrative cost, premiums charged by the carriers for coverage would still be unaffordable unless the tax credit was practically un-limited. None of the current tax credit proposals offers more than partial funding. Most have offered very small amounts of money, relative to the full premium needs of a fifty-year-old couple. Take another look at Figure 13.2, which shows average health care ex-penses by age. Look to see what these costs would be for each cat-egory. Double the costs for a couple.

The cash flow issues associated with a tax credit can also be a problem. The bureaucracy needed to determine eligibility and then produce sufficient and timely cash might create more hassles than most uninsured people are willing to deal with. Some people, par-ticularly higher-income uninsured who are already looking for cov-erage, would find pure tax credits to be a valuable tool. A lot of other people might find the process too complex and the dollars that are available inadequate to make coverage both accessible and affordable.

A Voucher Model, Like Medicare, Could Work for Many

So what can be done to make coverage more affordable to the point where we can cut the number of uninsured by at least half?

If we are willing to be bold and to learn from some pilot pro-grams that have already had some success, we can create a program that provides subsidized care, with low administrative costs, to low-income uninsured people. If the overall private health coverage marketplace for employers evolves to using some version of vouch-ers or defined contributions as the most common approach to pur-chasing group coverage, then that same group-based system could allow qualified low-income consumers to purchase care using sub-sidized vouchers provided by various state governments.

The vouchers could be used with various participating health plans in each market that are willing to sell voucher-friendly cov-erage options to their commercial clients.

Medicare already uses a similar system. The HMO program for Medicare now gives every Medicare recipient the equivalent of a voucher that each senior can use to buy coverage from a local participating health plan. Minnesota and Washington use that same system for their low-income uninsured populations today. So does Wisconsin. In those states, the government does the financial screening of individuals and issues the vouchers. Each uninsured person then selects a health plan. The uninsured people each pay a subsidized premium to the state based on their economic status. The state, in turn, pays a full premium to the health plan that the citizen selected.

That state-coordinated approach eliminates most of the administrative sales expenses and individual billing overhead costs that otherwise make nongroup commercial coverage so expensive. People could qualify for the subsidized coverage and vouchers simply by applying to the state. They could qualify for various subsidy levels based on their income level. In Minnesota, if those individuals are unhappy with the plan they chose, they simply take their voucher to another plan. The percentage of uninsured in Minnesota has been cut to under two-thirds of the national rate.

Using vouchers for low-income uninsured people to buy health plan coverage is an approach that truly creates a public-private partnership. Medicare pioneered the model of a public-private partnership by allowing individual Medicare recipients to select health plans in a competitive marketplace. Extending a similar model to the low-income uninsured could remove a major burden to coverage and help eliminate the wasteful administrative expenses of the individual insurance marketplace.

If the cafeteria model of benefit choice is extended to the new low-income, subsidized coverage program (as opposed to the usual one-size-fits-all comprehensive benefit approach used for Medicaid) and some benefit options are included in the package, then individuals would be able to make their own benefit choices based on their own needs.

There are some challenging actuarial issues to be resolved before that model can be widely offered, but experiments in private coverage involving choice show that these issues can be resolved.

How Do We Keep Employers from Abandoning Coverage?

A major concern of policymakers is that many employers that now offer subsidized coverage to their employees may choose to pull back on that financial support if an alternative, subsidized federal coverage program is made available to employees. That concern could be mitigated somewhat by antidiscrimination laws that would keep employers from excluding some employees from group coverage.

Perhaps the easiest way of preventing employers from abandoning coverage would be to enact "pay or play" laws that require all employers to make a contribution toward health care coverage for each employee. A number of these proposals are being considered. Coupled with real market reform, they might have a broad and positive impact on the uninsured population.

Minnesota does not allow low-income people to enroll in the subsidized plan if their employer offers group coverage. That provision will have to be amended if we want to cover the 47 percent of the uninsured who turn down group coverage now because it's unaffordable.

A better model might be to give employers a tax break for covering their low-income employees so long as the net result of the tax break is to increase the total number of people being covered without reducing current employer contributions. A goal in that case would be to have the low-income employees with an out-of-pocket expense that runs parallel to the premiums paid by individuals who enroll in the state-subsidized programs.

Whereas tax credits may be too little and too late for most low-income individuals, they could be a major tool for employers. The government could allow employers to receive direct-tax credits for providing coverage to employees at very low income levels—perhaps at 150 percent of the U.S. poverty level. Those tax credits could help the employer continue to subsidize group coverage. The administrative cost levels of group coverage could be contained. Done well, all members of staff would benefit.

These programs, properly executed, could significantly reduce the number of permanently uninsured working Americans. At a time when the number of employed but uninsured persons is otherwise going to grow significantly because of health care cost pressures, we should act now to extend coverage as broadly as we can.

Community Clinics Have a Major Role to Play

For the remaining uninsured, its time to revisit the concept of expanding government subsidies to well-planned, carefully managed community clinics. Particularly in some large urban areas, an expanded system of nonprofit or even government-run clinics could be a major gap filler for people who make too much money for Medicaid and too little to buy even subsidized vouchers. For major segments of our uninsured population, there probably isn't any insurance-based market model that will work. This is particularly true in areas where the uninsured are low-income people whose immigration status is a bit unclear, causing them to avoid more formal programs of any kind. For those populations, we very much need a safety net network of care sites that provide very low-cost care to all patients, regardless of coverage. Those clinics, strategically located in both inner cities and rural high-parity areas, could do a lot of good for a major segment of our uninsured population.

Staff Community Clinics with Subsidized Professionals

It's time to rethink our community clinic strategy. We need more of those care sites as soon as possible. How would we fund and staff these clinics? To alleviate our long-term health care staffing needs, as well as staff the new community care sites, we might want to issue a whole new round of health professional scholarships—funding complete education for qualified students in nursing, medical technology, and medicine—with a requirement that each graduate student work for a designated number of years (at a good level of pay) in those care sites. If those programs are well designed, there will be a significant improvement in care for our lower-income, uninsured population, and those sites will give us the candidates we need so badly for our long-term care needs.

We've resisted expanding our nation's "free" clinics for a number of years. In some settings, that leaves a massive void that will never be filled, in a time of shrinking health care human resources, by pure market forces. When the suburban hospitals and clinics pay top dollar, how else will we lure qualified caregivers to the heart of our cities where they are so badly needed?

Tax credits will not create care in Watts or East Oakland. A U.S. health corps might. It's worth designing.

17

Training Tomorrow's Caregivers and
Reengineering Care Delivery

A merica can change its insurance laws overnight. It takes over a decade to train a doctor. It takes four years to train a baccalaureate-degreed nurse, and many students take five years to complete the program. If we want to have a sufficient number of health care professionals in all the right categories of care ten years from now, we need to be planning today to meet those needs.

Given the current levels of enrollment in the various nursing, medical technologist, and health care support professional schools, it's clear that we are headed for a major shortfall. Miracles won't happen without the staff necessary to make them happen.

Without a plan for correcting those problems, market forces will act on their own. Shortages of any needed product create high prices. Massive shortages of health care workers will result in ever increasing pay levels for the workers available. Ultimately, those pay increases will make the caregiving professions attractive enough to lure a whole new generation into providing care. That whole process will take many years, however, and it will push health care costs up at an even faster rate than they are rising today. A proactive approach to training and staffing would be more affordable for us all in the long run. The approach outlined in Chapter Sixteen—to give full scholarships to needed health care students in exchange for several years of practice in a low-income clinic setting—may help. It's worth considering.

Simply increasing the number of available workers will help, but an equally important strategy needs to be built around redesigning the health care delivery system to make the whole process more efficient in its use of resources. We also need to focus on the demand for care: improving health where possible rather than simply extending care to more people.

To accomplish those goals, we need to be taking a hard look at the processes and systems used to deliver care today. Education, medical research, and expert levels of systems engineering and reengineering all need to be aimed at improving the quality of care, improving the efficacy of care delivery, guaranteeing ongoing access to care, and bringing health care delivery approaches into the new century.

This will be an entirely new effect in health care. At this point, there is no structural agenda aimed at meeting those goals. The whole topic of care reengineering is not on the table for America's caregivers.

We also need a much more aggressive set of research projects to determine how to better align the health care delivery system to prevent diseases. We also need research to figure out how best to treat patients with chronic conditions. Those patients will soon be consuming the majority of our nation's health care resources, and we are not treating them either efficiently or well. Some of the more progressive health plans and medical groups are now building systematic disease management programs for chronic care patients. Aside from those efforts, however, the standard health care delivery nonsystem is ignoring those important issues altogether.

In other words, our strategy for resolving the upcoming shortage of health care workers needs those major components: (1) train more workers, (2) reengineer care processes to make available workers more efficient, and (3) focus on preventing the disease situations that are increasing the demand for care.

Our country has no master strategy for the training of health care professionals. We don't even have meaningful projections of our future needs for most categories of health care workers. No one is figuring out how many nurses, technicians, care aides, and physicians we will need for the next five to twenty years. No one in Washington or in the various state houses is studying exactly how to recruit or develop new caregivers. That's a mistake. We need to upgrade and update our thinking about the most appropriate ways of training health care professionals and put those programs in place as quickly as possible.

Simultaneously, we need major government support for pilot programs and research programs designed to reengineer care. We are still, almost without exception, using the entire array of caregivers exactly as they were used in 1980. Computers have entered our world since then. New technologies and communication tools exist. New monitoring tools exist. Amazingly, those tools have had relatively minimal application in health care. They have not caused care in hospitals, clinics, or nursing homes to be reengineered in any significant way.

We Need Unfettered Test Sites to Redefine Care Jobs Around Patient Needs

No one involved in front-line care currently has the money, time, or perspective to spend on reengineering care. The old joke about being too focused on the alligators to spend time draining the swamp sums up the situation in health care today. A vast amount of money is being spent on new medical technology, but almost no money is available to figure out the optimal uses of that technology. The federal government could play a major role here. Someone needs to create a resource that will allow qualified test sites to rethink care delivery in the light of modern tools, modern technology, and modern needs. Funded test sites could look creatively at the most productive use of all categories of health care professionals.

We need to focus first on the needs of patients and then work backward to design systems that meet those needs. The current systems are designed largely around the needs of caregivers. As we move into the twenty-first century, the new systems ought to be built around the needs of patients. As we build those new system designs, we need to be flexible and innovative.

To do that, we will need test sites that are freed from a number of the constraints and fairly rigid role definitions and work rules that have been built into the current system by laws, contracts, guilds, and custom. Ideally, these test sites could figure out what optimal patient care would look like and then make job assignments to the caregivers based on that optimal model. That process would undoubtedly require some blurring of the boundary lines between categories of caregivers as opposed to today's fairly rigid castes of caregivers. Test sites would need clear authority from lawmakers, medical leaders, and union officials to redesign the role of the pharmacist, technician, doctor, and nurse, all in the best interest of patients.

This will not be easy to do. If we do redefine roles of caregivers, then in some cases, rigid work rules built into union contracts will need to be made more flexible. Rigid divisions of authority and scope of practice built into licensing laws will need to be made more open to new science and new potentialities.

This is not a call for licensing anarchy or work role chaos. The reengineering pilot programs need to be conducted under the strictest oversight and quality monitoring to be sure that patients benefit and the highest-quality standards are followed. That will cost money. Reengineering, monitoring, and oversight are all expensive. That's where government grants could help. The challenge, then, will be to avoid having the system micromanaged by policymakers far from the front lines of care.

Many would advocate that we let the private marketplace somehow independently achieve these kinds of innovations. Usually that's a preferred model. Health care, however, is already so constrained by the government, which sets the work rules for all caregivers, that only the government can create the freedom and funding needed to make these pilots work. The private health care marketplace is too controlled by laws and contracts even to attempt some of the most potentially useful of those patient-centered workforce redesign experiments. In other words, because the government sets the work rules for all caregivers, it needs to be a partner in liberating the system from those rules.

A well-designed operational research program for hospitals and related care delivery systems could move health care delivery forward. Without that effort, the inefficiencies of the old system will be hard to dislodge. Given today's health care cost environment, we need to do better.

Would reengineering of the system make a difference? Kaiser Permanente of Colorado is experimenting with an approach that adds clinical pharmacists to the care team. The pharmacists improve the quality of drug therapy by educating physicians and patients about national guidelines, helping to avoid adverse drug reactions, and consulting with surgical teams in advance of procedures on patients on anticoagulant medications. For patients on a high-risk drug like warfarin, this approach has resulted in an 81 percent reduction in major bleeding, reduced hospital admissions, and the saving of many lives. These results were obtained only because the system of delivering care was redesigned in an improved, collaborative way.

Build the New System Around Best Care

As we run various pilot programs to figure out the best uses of our health care resources, we also need to be redesigning our approach to all levels of care. Chronic care is a good place to start. We have huge opportunities for both care improvement and cost savings relative to chronic care patients. But we haven't spent enough time as a country designing the best systems of care for those patients.

The government should be investing heavily in disease management research for chronic care. Almost all current government-subsidized medical research focuses on the cutting edges of care: the new technologies, drugs, and procedures that deliver miraculous outcomes for patients suffering from acute conditions. Most medical researchers focus on this kind of research because it's the kind that earns grants in today's academic environment. It's hard to persuade anyone to do unfunded research. But if we decide as a nation to create a health care policy that has, as a major goal, improving the overall delivery of care, then we should fund solid research aimed at improving care. We need research that tells us not only what the optimal behaviors are for people with diabetes but also what the very best ways are of getting them to choose the kinds of behaviors that will measurably reduce the rate of diabetic complications.

We need further research into preventing preterm births. What do we need to do to reduce preterm births to half of current levels? We need research that identifies optimal approaches for helping depressed people. What kinds of care systems and care approaches will identify depressed people earlier, help them cope more effectively, and end the cycles of both chemical imbalance and despair that too often end in surrender and suicide?

Depression is almost always treated as an episode of care, with a single caregiver providing intermittent services to a single patient. Is that the best model? What are the measurable results of that model? Does a team-based model that links primary care physicians to mental health professionals for the care of a given patient offer better outcomes?

Some very smart people say yes, but we don't know if they are right, because, in the absence of an overall national health care policy aimed at systematically improving health, those experiments aren't being done and those research efforts aren't currently funded. So inadequate care continues. New approaches are unfounded and untested.

What research is being done to help the children of divorce avoid psychological damage? We know that depressed children tend to be less healthy and use more health care resources. Why not deal with that issue proactively? What research is being done into systematic approaches that will help those children do better in the years after their parents' divorce? Whole areas of important learning are not even being explored.

Pure research into molecules and technology should also continue to be a major component of the federally funded research agenda for this country. We haven't put much emphasis on that issue in this book because we know that research in those areas will continue at warp speed. It's the American way. Our medical scientists will outdo themselves year after year with better machines, more sophisticated technologies, and better surgical techniques. Those developments will be financially rewarded by the American system of health care financing. The best inventors and technologists will get rich, or richer, treating disease, fixing problems.

The real problem is that no one gets rich inventing approaches or delivering care that prevents disease or avoids problems. Up to this point, proactively improving health hasn't been very profitable, so it gets little or no attention from health care capitalists.

This will change somewhat when gene analysis becomes an industry that can make a lot of money by helping people anticipate health problems. Proactive imaging approaches may soon be able to help people get a jump-start on avoiding various kinds of heart crisis or system problems. Those approaches to disease prevention will receive a disproportionate amount of publicity and funding compared to other disease prevention approaches.

The reason is that someone can make a lot of money by doing a gene scan or a baseline MRI scan—a lot more money than anyone can make advising people to stop smoking, lose weight, or increase physical activity levels.

Follow the dollars. That's why, if we really want the system to focus on best care, we probably need government-funded programs to initiate efforts and prove value in those areas.

We now need an operational research agenda targeted at improving the ground-level delivery of care for the people in this country who have the common and chronic diseases of everyday life. If we don't improve our care for those diseases in systematic ways, then the costs associated with those diseases will continue to explode.

The system will not cure itself. The problems of the system need to be diagnosed and then treated.

The ultimate alternative to a practical redesign of the system, sadly, will be a cost explosion that results in government intervention, care rationing, massive cost shifting, and the probable emergence of a two-class system, with the wealthy still getting great care and everyone else being treated in an understaffed, underfunded, undermotivated, and inconsistently effective nonsystem of care.

We can do better. But only if we try. What would it look like if we tried?

. . . .

18

A Call to Action

A highly respected Minnesotan labor leader was looking at the health care cost increases his union locals were facing. He saw insurance premium increases so high that they were dwarfing his workers' painfully negotiated wage increases.

Looking at the care utilization levels of the insurance plans, he said, "What's costing us right now is an epidemic of care. If this keeps up, this epidemic of care will bankrupt us just as fast as an epidemic of polio. We want the best care—but we need to figure out how to get it for less money."

He was accurate in his diagnosis. We are facing an epidemic of care—some might say an avalanche of care. We are seeing new drugs, new technologies, and new techniques, all being used by an aging, out-of-shape, increasingly demanding, and increasingly sophisticated patient population. That epidemic of care is being perversely fueled by a set of provider economic incentives focused exclusively on units of care and volumes of services, with little or no reward going to anyone in the entire system for efforts to reduce disease, improve safety, or produce needed care at a higher level of efficiency.

What can we do about that situation?

We can start by demanding a focus on evidence-based medicine and medical best practices. As long as we're spending more than a trillion dollars per year on health care, we should be getting the best care.

. . . . .

In every major area of care—cancer, heart disease, diabetes, kidney failure—the levels of caregiver inconsistency in this country are so great as to be almost beyond belief. When best practices can literally cut the rate of premature births in half, then we ought to be ashamed of a nonsystem that lets so many babies be born so prematurely that their lives are in danger and they are in misery from the moment of birth.

We ought to be ashamed of a system that lets two times too many people go through the hell of a congestive heart failure crisis. We ought to be entirely unaccepting of care delivery that lets stroke victims who could be rehabilitated end up with permanent crippling incapacities and functional impairments.

The issue of care inconsistency and the need to improve the quality of care should be understood by buyers, patients, and consumers and dealt with systematically by America's care systems and health plans. We're past the point where the status quo should be tolerated in most of those areas.

Accountability

We're at the point where consumers should start getting information about care system and caregiver performance. Standards of care like those created by the American Diabetes Association should exist for every major disease area. Health plans and specialty organizations should let the public know which providers do well in adhering to those standards and which do poorly. When miracles are available, the public deserves to know exactly which local care systems are and are not making those miracles happen.

Miracles Cost Money

We need widespread recognition that medical miracles generally cost money. The news media, health plans, community leaders, and health system leaders all need to do a much better job of exploring and explaining both the cost and value of today's incredible toolbox of medical miracles.

We all need to understand the value equation because we're all paying the costs through our premiums, and we all deserve to know exactly why our premiums are increasing.

As part of the recognition of value, we need to reengineer America's health insurance benefit levels. People need protection against the unaffordable costs of care, but the current system of insurance typically goes one step further and insulates most consumers entirely from any and all costs of care. That total insulation keeps most people from being directly involved in determining whether various care approaches are worth the money they cost. That's a mistake that leads to wasted and inappropriately utilized health care resources.

A more sophisticated benefit approach would involve more cost sharing by patients, with the new cost-sharing features focused primarily on various elective levels of care. (Increasing copayments for multiple unsuccessful attempts at creating fertility might be one example of an area where benefit redesign might be useful and good public policy.)

A combination of cost-shared benefit sets for consumers and a heavy reliance on evidence-based care for physicians has the potential to improve care significantly while using health care dollars more appropriately. Add to that mixture increasingly discerning and sophisticated Internet-savvy consumers who have access to far more information about their care and their caregivers than in the past, and we will move a long way down the road to a more responsible care system. Each disease ought to have its own credible information infrastructure. Ideally, consumers with diabetes should be able to go to the Internet and learn about diabetic best care, diabetic care treatment options, and the relative performance of local caregivers who treat diabetes.

A pipe dream? A futurist wish list? Not at all. Go to the HealthPartners Web site now (www.healthpartners.com) and see care protocols for people with diabetes created by the best diabetes experts in the country. Then click over to see how various providers in this network have done on diabetic care follow-up. You can even check on outcomes, like the relative success of various caregivers in controlling blood sugar levels for their diabetic patients. The reporting we are calling for isn't a policy wonk wish list. It's happening now. But it isn't happening in very many places. That needs to change.

We are also at the point where a true restructuring of the health insurance market can finally be achieved. A marketplace that publishes caregiver performance data and fosters informed consumer choices will enable the best care systems and the best caregivers to be rewarded for their achievements and added value. A performance-based marketplace in health care is long overdue and finally possible, thanks to the work of inspired physician leaders like John Wennberg, Gordon Mosser, and Don Berwick, to name just a few. Before now, buyers couldn't insist on a quality-based marketplace because the tools to create that marketplace did not exist. They do now, so it's time for sophisticated buyers to make the kinds of choices that will evolve health care into the next generation of value. It's also time for the government to encourage the kind of market reform that will result in informed, value-based decisions by consumers and patients relative to both insurance coverage and care.

Enact New "Rules of the Road"

If we are to have a health insurance system that is accessible to all and more stable than the current one, we will need to enact some important reforms. These "rules of the road" should benefit all who are involved with the system: consumers, caregivers, plans, employers, and regulators. As we have stated previously, we favor expanding coverage through the employer-based system. But the current voluntary system allows many employers—even some very large ones—to avoid paying coverage. And the current approach to competition among health plans does not promote affordable coverage for all.

Eventually, we will need to consider adopting a program like the one that Hawaii has now: by law, most employers are required to provide health insurance to their employees. If we take that direction, we will need other reforms so the system works to the benefit of all—for example:

- A defined-benefit package that would be made available by health plans

- Fair rules on offering and pricing the benefit package so that those are who are sicker can still afford to buy health insurance

- Rules of competition that encourage health plans and health care professionals to provide the highest quality at an affordable cost

Because many people are not linked to an employer, we will continue to need publicly sponsored or subsidized programs to assist lower-income people in getting necessary health coverage, and we will need funding and innovative programs to support inner-city and rural health services for underserved populations.

Automation of Key Physician Support Tools Is Absolutely Essential

Probably the single most important tool we need now to create the infrastructure foundation that will allow every other value improvement strategy to happen is the computer. Specifically, that key tool is an automated medical record, available to the doctor and patient in the exam room at the point of care. Without that tool, it takes years to implement each and every change in medical science. Without that tool, consistency around best practices is almost impossible to achieve. Without that tool, medical research takes ten times as long and costs ten times as much money.

Without that tool, accountability is, at best, based on indirect information and incomplete data. Without that tool, excess administrative costs continue to eat a hole in the health care dollar. It's time for health care to join the rest of the professions in using the computer to directly improve performance. That will be a revolutionary development, and once it has been done well, we will all wonder how we ever functioned without it.

Let's Get Best Health in Return for Our Dollars

Health care will be changing dramatically over the next several years. Nothing on the horizon now will reduce care costs. Just about everything—every drug, technique, and piece of technology—being developed will improve care while directly and immediately adding costs.

We need to be realistic about that fact. If the percentage of GNP focused on health does climb to 20 or even 25 percent, that's not necessarily a catastrophe if what we get in return is much greater functionality, better lives, and best health. But if what we get in return is just an extremely expensive extension of our current, too-often dysfunctional nonsystem, with a myopic resource focus and emphasis on after-the-fact heroic medicine, costly damage control, and crisis management tools, then the system will implode from its own cost burden. The consequences for our economy could be dire. The cost burden of inconsistent and unaccountable care will force millions of people to lose coverage entirely. Ultimately, the government would have to step in to impose controls of some kind. Those controls in every other country with a government-based health insurance system for care delivery have resulted in the direct—and often severe—rationing of care based on government budget constraints.

Let's not let that happen here. Let's make our system work and generate enough value to be an investment we make in good health for all of us.

The tools finally exist. We just have to make the strategic decision as a nation to use them.

Notes

• •

Introduction

1. S. Heffler and others, "Health Spending Projections for 2001–2011: The Latest Outlook," *Health Affairs* (Mar.–Apr. 2002): 207–218.

2. S. Altman, *Uncontrolled Health Inflation: The Growing Crisis in the U.S. Health Care System* (Washington, D.C.: Alliance for Health Reform, 2002). [www.allhealth.org/recent/audio_08-02-02/Altman.pdf].

3. Kaiser Family Foundation and Health Research and Educational Trust, "Employer Health Benefits: 2002 Annual Survey" (Menlo Park, Calif.: Kaiser Family Foundation, 2002); Joel E. Miller, *A Perfect Storm: The Confluence of Forces Affecting Health Care Coverage* (Washington, D.C.: National Coalition on Health Care, Nov. 2001).

4. R. J. Mills, *Health Insurance Coverage: 2001* (Washington, D.C.: U.S. Government Printing Office, 2002).

5. American Medical Association, "CPT (Current Procedural Terminology)," Oct. 14, 2001. [http://www.ama-assn.org/ama/pub/printcat/3113.html].

6. American Association for Retired People, *Beyond 50: A Report to the Nation on Trends in Health Security* (Washington, D.C.: American Association for Retired People, May 2002).

7. M. I. Harris and R. C. Eastman, "Early Detection of Undiagnosed Non-Insulin-Dependent Diabetes Mellitus," *Journal of the American Medical Association* 276 (1996): 1261–1262.

Chapter One

1. HealthPartners, "Annual Cost for Premature Infants," internal report (Minneapolis: HealthPartners, Mar. 15, 2001).

2. HealthPartners, "Thalamic Stimulation for Essential Tremor or Parkinson's Disease," internal report (Minneapolis: HealthPartners, Mar. 2, 2001).

3. HealthPartners, "Stereotactic Radiosurgery Gamma Knife," internal report (Minneapolis: HealthPartners, Mar. 2, 2001).

4. HealthPartners, "Lung Volume Reduction Surgery," internal report (Minneapolis: HealthPartners, Mar. 2, 2001).

5. HealthPartners, "Transplants," internal report (Minneapolis: HealthPartners, Mar. 2, 2001).

6. HealthPartners, "Islet Cell Transplantation," internal report (Minneapolis: HealthPartners, Mar. 2, 2001).

7. Ron Winslow, "New Heart Stents Deliver Drugs to Blockage Site," *Wall Street Journal*, Jan. 12, 2001.

8. Winslow, "New Heart Stents Deliver Drugs to Blockage Site."

9. Lynn Yoffee, "Restenosis: Drug-Coated Stents Prevent Blockages in the Long Term," *Heart Disease Weekly*, Apr. 28, 2002.

10. Winslow, "New Heart Stents Deliver Drugs to Blockage Site."

11. *2000 Drug Topics Red Book* (Montvale, N.J.: Medical Economics Company, 2000), p. 577.

12. *2000 Drug Topics Red Book*, p. 492.

13. *2000 Drug Topics Red Book*, p. 392.

14. "Managing Antibiotic Resistance," *New England Journal of Medicine*, Dec. 28, 2000, p. 1961.

15. Michael Chernew, A. Mark Fendrick, and Richard A. Hirth, "Managed Care and Medical Technology: Implications for Cost Growth," *Health Affairs* 16:2 (Mar.–Apr. 1997): 196–206.

16. Barney J. Feder, "Scalpel! Clamp! . . . Hemopure?" *New York Times*, Mar. 4, 2001, p. 1.

17. J. Bruce Moseley and others, "A Controlled Trial of Arthroscopic Surgery for Osteoarthritis of the Knee," *New England Journal of Medicine*, July 11, 2002, pp. 81–88.

Chapter Two

1. Institute of Medicine, *To Err Is Human: Building a Safer Health System* (Washington, D.C.: National Academy of Sciences, 1999), p. 1.

2. Mark R. Chassin, "Is Health Care Ready for Six Sigma Quality?" *Milbank Quarterly* 76:4 (1998). [http://www.Milbank.org/quarterly/764featchas.html].

3. Bill Runciman, "Protecting the Patient" (rate based on presentation to the International Federation of Health Plans, Cairns, Australia, Sept. 2000). [http://www.hfh.com/proceedings/08_protect_patient.doc.html].

4. Institute of Medicine, *To Err Is Human*, p. 42.

5. Jennifer Steinhauer, "So, the Tumor Is on the Left, Right?" *New York Times*, Apr. 1, 2001. [http://www.nytimes.com/2001/04/01/health/01SURG.html].

6. Joint Commission on Accreditation of Health Care Organizations, *Sentinel Event Alert*, Dec. 5, 2001. [http://www.jcaho.org/about+us/news+letters/sentinel+event+alert/print/sea_24.htm].

7. Steinhauer, "So, the Tumor Is on the Left, Right?"

8. Steinhauer, "So, the Tumor Is on the Left, Right?"

9. J. Skinner and J. E. Wennberg, "How Much Is Enough? Efficiency and Medicare Spending in the Last Six Months of Life," in D. M. Cutler (ed.), *The Changing Hospital Industry: Comparing Not-for-Profit and For-Profit Institutions* (Chicago: University of Chicago Press, 2000), pp. 169–193. J. E. Wennberg, "Excerpt from *Dealing with Medical Practice Variations: A Proposal for Action*," *Health Affairs* 3:2 (1984): 6–32. J. E. Wennberg, "On the Appropriateness of Small-Area Analysis for Cost Containment," *Health Affairs* (Winter 1996): 164–167. J. E. Wennberg, "Outcomes Research, Cost Containment, and the Fear of Health Care Rationing," *New England*

Journal of Medicine 323:17 (1990): 1202–1204. J. E. Wennberg, J. L. Freeman, and W. J. Culp, "Are Hospital Services Rationed in New Haven or Over-Utilized in Boston?" *Lancet* 1:8543 (1987): 1185–1189. Elliott S. Fisher and others, "Associations Among Hospital Capacity, Utilization, and Mortality of U.S. Medicare Beneficiaries, Controlling for Sociodemographic Factors," *Health Services Research*, Feb. 1, 2000, p. 1351.

10. Institute of Medicine, *Crossing the Quality Chasm: A New Health System for the Twenty-First Century* (Washington, D.C.: National Academy of Sciences, 2001).

11. American Heart Association, "Heart Attacks and Angina Statistics," 2002. [http://www.americanheart.org/Heart_and_Stroke_A_Z_Guide/has.html].

12. HealthPartners, "Congestive Heart Failure," internal report (Minneapolis: HealthPartners, Jan. 27, 2003).

13. National Institute of Diabetes and Digestive and Kidney Diseases, *Diabetes Statistics* (Bethesda, Md.: National Institutes of Health, Oct. 1995).

14. Ali H. Mokdad and others, "Diabetes Trends in the US: 1990–1998," *Diabetes Care* 23:9 (Sept. 2000): 1278–1283.

15. Mokdad and others, "Diabetes Trends in the US."

16. Patrick J. O'Connor and others, "Care of Adults with Type 2 Diabetes Mellitus," *Journal of Family Practice* 47:5 (suppl.) (1998): S13-S21.

17. K. L. Nichol and others, "The Efficacy and Cost Effectiveness of Vaccination Against Influenza Among Elderly Persons Living in the Community," *New England Journal of Medicine*, Sept. 22, 1994, pp. 778–784.

18. Unpublished study, forthcoming.

19. Midwest Business Group on Health, *Reducing the Costs of Poor Quality Health Care Through Responsible Purchasing Leadership* (Chicago: Midwest Business Group on Health, June 2002).

20. E-mail communication with Karen Patrias, reference librarian, National Library of Medicine, Apr. 27, 2001.

21. Laura Landro, "Health Advocates Seek Guidelines That Stick to Proven Treatments," *Wall Street Journal*, May 11, 2001, p. B1.

22. A. O. Berg, "Variations Among Family Physicians' Management Strategies for Lower Urinary Tract Infection in Women: A Report from The Washington Family Physicians Collective Research Network," *Journal of the American Board of Family Practices*, (Sept.–Oct. 1991): 327–330.

23. HealthPartners, "Health Clinical Quality Profile," internal report (Minneapolis: HealthPartners, Mar. 21, 2001).

24. HealthPartners, "HealthPartners Cardiology Specialist Pilot Patient Results, 1999," internal report (Minneapolis: HealthPartners, 1999).

25. HealthPartners, "HealthPartners Cardiology Specialist Pilot PCP Results," internal report (Minneapolis: HealthPartners, 1999).

26. HealthPartners, "HealthPartners HEDIS 2002 Report," internal report (Minneapolis: HealthPartners, 2002), p. 18, based on 2001 dates of service.

27. HealthPartners, "HealthPartners HEDIS 2002 Report."

28. HealthPartners, "HealthPartners Medical Clinics Clinical Indicators Report," internal report (Minneapolis: HealthPartners, Aug. 1996).

Chapter Three

1. HealthPartners, "Claims Distribution," 2002 internal report (Minneapolis: HealthPartners, 2002).

2. M. Pauly, A. Percy, and B. Herring, "Individual Versus Job-Based Health Insurance: Weighing the Pros and Cons," *Health Affairs* 18:6 (Nov.–Dec. 1999): 28–44. The authors estimate that administrative costs are about 5 percent of premium for the largest groups, 20 to 25 percent for the smallest groups (fewer than twenty-five employees), and 30 percent in the nongroup market.

Chapter Four

1. Nancy E. Mayo and others, "Waiting Time for Breast Cancer Surgery in Quebec," *Canadian Medical Association Journal* 164 (2001): 1133–1138.

2. "NHS Keeps Patients Waiting for Longer," Nov. 14, 2000. [www. thetimes.co.uk/article/].

3. Sarah Lyall, "In Britain's Health Service, Sick Itself, Cancer Care Is Dismal," *New York Times*, Feb. 10, 2000, A1.

4. Richard G. A. Feachem, Neelam K. Sekhri, and Karen L. White, "Getting More for Their Dollar: A Comparison of the NHS with California's Kaiser Permanente," *British Medical Journal* 324 (2002): 135–143.

5. Organization for Economic Cooperation and Development, *OECD Health Data 2002*, 4th ed. (Paris: Organization for Economic Cooperation and Development, 2002).

6. Lyall, "In Britain's Health Service, Sick Itself," p. A1.

7. "Number of NHS Patients Treated Privately Soars, Boost to Private Sector," *NewsEdge WorkGroups*, Feb. 20, 2001. [http://workgroups. newsedge.com/].

8. "Daily Mail/In Need of a Hospital Bed? Try Germany," *NewsEdge WorkGroups*, Feb. 9, 2001. [http://workgroups.newsedge.com/].

9. "Scotland on Sunday/NHS Waiting Times Surge," *NewsEdge WorkGroups*, Feb. 20, 2001. ([http://workgroups.newsedge.com/].

10. "Canadians with Medical Needs Follow Their Doctors South," *Wall Street Journal*, Mar. 5, 1999, p. A15.

11. Julian Beltrame, "To Ease Crisis in Health Care, Canadians Eye Private Sector," *Wall Street Journal*, Apr. 19, 2000, p. B1.

12. William McArthur, "Memo to Al Gore: Canadian Medicine Isn't Cheap or Effective," *Wall Street Journal*, Jan. 28, 2000, p. A19.

13. "Report's Denial of Healthcare Crisis Prevents True Reform/Fraser Institute," NewsEdge WorkGroups, Jan. 26, 2001. [http://workgroups. newsedge.com/display_p.asp?doc_id=Nea0125185.900].

14. Personal communication.

Chapter Five

1. George C. Halvorson, "Health Plan's Strategic Responses to a Changing Marketplace," *Health Affairs* 18 (Mar.–Apr. 1999): 28.

2. Henry J. Kaiser Family Foundation, *Prescription Drug Trends* (Menlo Park, Calif.: Henry J. Kaiser Family Foundation, July 2000), exhibit 4.1.

Chapter Six

1. *Physician Compensation and Production Survey, 2000 Report Based on 1999 Data* (Englewood, Colo.: Medical Group Management Association, 2000), p. 11.

2. The 1996 acute care hospital costs per day were $1,128 in the United States, $489 in Canada, and $320 in the United Kingdom. Organization for Economic Cooperation and Development, *OECD Health Data 1998* (Paris: Organization for Economic Cooperation and Development, 1998).

3. HealthPartners Pharmacy Department, internal memo, Dec. 4, 2000.

4. John Ewoldt, "Don't Let the Price of Pills Make You Sick—Try These Remedies," *Star Tribune*, Apr. 26, 2001, p. E1.

5. Stephen S. Hall, "The Claritin Effect: Prescription for Profit," New York Times on the Web, Mar. 11, 2001. [file://D:<\ \ >New%20York%20Times%20Search.htm].

6. U.S. Food and Drug Administration, *Direct-to-Consumer Advertising of Prescription Drugs: Preliminary Patient Survey Results* (Washington, D.C.: U.S. Government Printing Office, May 10, 2002). [http://www.fda.gov/cder/ddmac/DTCnational2002a/sld001.html].

7. Crain Communications, "Legislators May Move on DTC Drug Advertising," NewsEdge WorkGroups, Apr. 9, 2001. [http://workgroups.newsedge.com/display_p.asp?doc_id=Nec0406302.6rn].

8. Howard Bell, "Drug Prices in Search of a Fix," *Minnesota Medicine: A Journal of Clinical and Health Affairs* 84 (Jan. 2001): 26.

9. Bell, "Drug Prices in Search of a Fix," p. 26.

10. Todd Melby, "Directly to Consumers," *Metro Doctors: Journal of the Hennepin and Ramsey Medical Societies* 2:2 (Mar.–Apr. 2000): 13.

11. *2000 Drug Topics Red Book* (Montvale, N.J.: Medical Economics Company, 2000), p. 531.

12. U.S. Food and Drug Administration, Center for Drug Evaluation and Research, Division Director Memorandum NDA: 21–087, Oct. 25, 1999. [http://www.fda.gov/cder/drug/infopage/tamiflu/directormemo.htm].

13. *2000 Drug Topics Red Book*, p. 393.

14. SmithKline Beecham Pharmaceuticals, *Prescribing Information for Selected Products* (Philadelphia: SmithKline Beecham Pharmaceuticals, Sept. 1999), p. 10.

15. Hall, "The Claritin Effect."

16. Crain Communications, "Legislators May Move on DTC Drug Advertising."

17. "DTC Drug Ads Backlash," *Health Market Survey Friday Report*, Mar. 30, 2001. [healthnews@starpower.net].

18. Henry J. Kaiser Family Foundation, *Prescription Drug Trends* (Menlo Park, Calif.: Henry J. Kaiser Family Foundation, July 2000), exhibit 2.3.

19. Kaiser Family Foundation, *Prescription Drug Trends*, exhibit 2.3.

20. David Noonan, "Why Drugs Cost So Much," Special Report, *Newsweek*, Sept. 25, 2000.

21. "Prescription Drug Prices: Are We Getting Our Money's Worth?" *Medical Benefits*, 7 (March 15, 1990): 1.

Chapter Seven

1. "Cyberchondriacs Update," Harris Poll 19, Apr. 18, 2001. [http://www.harrisinteractive.com/harris_poll/index.asp?PID-229].

2. John Fry and Gerald Sandler, *Common Diseases*, 5th ed. (Norwell, Mass.: Kluwer, 1993), pp. 31, 261, 271, 318.

3. A. O. Berg, "Variations Among Family Physicians' Management Strategies for Lower Urinary Tract Infection in Women: A Report from The Washington Family Physicians Collective Research Network," *Journal of the American Board of Family Practices*, (Sept.–Oct. 1991): 327–330.

4. "Grants from NIH and Industry for U.S. Clinical Trials to Exceed $4 Billion in 2000 According to CenterWatch Research," Center-Watch Clinical Trials Listing Service, Nov. 2000. [http://www.centerwatch.com/pressreleases.html].

Chapter Eight

1. U.S. Department of Health and Human Services, Health Resources and Services Administration, *Projected Supply, Demand, and Shortages of Registered Nurses: 2000–2020* (Washington, D.C.: U.S. Government Printing Office, July 2002).

2. Dave Carpenter, "Going . . . Going . . . Gone?" *Hospitals and Health Networks* 74:6 (June 2000): 32.

3. U.S. Department of Health and Human Services, *Projected Supply, Demand, and Shortages of Registered Nurses: 2000–2020*.

4. Linda H. Aiken and others, "Hospital Nurse Staffing and Patient Mortality, Nurse Burnout, and Job Dissatisfaction," *Journal of the America Medical Association*, Oct. 23–30, 2002, pp. 1987–1993.

5. "Where Have All the Nurses Gone?" *HealthcareBusiness* (June 2000). [http://www.healthcarebusiness.com/archives/healthcarebusiness/0600/feature.html].

6. American Medical Association Council on Medical Service, *The Growing Nursing Shortage in the United States* (Chicago: American Medical Association, June 2001).

7. Mary Chris Jaklevic and Ed Lovern, "A Nursing Code Blue," *Modern Healthcare*, Dec. 11, 2000, pp. 42–44.

8. Jennifer Steinhauer, "Shortage of Health Care Workers Keeps Growing," *New York Times*, Dec. 25, 2000, p. A.

9. "Recruitment and Retention," *Nursing Executive Watch*, Feb. 2, 2001, p. 6.

10. Martin, Fletcher, *Nursing and Allied Health Care Annual Compensation and Benefits Report* (Irving, Tex.: Martin, Fletcher, Apr. 2001).

11. "Nurse Shortage Growing Worse," *USA Today*, Aug. 3, 2000. [http://www.usatoday.com/life/health/hcare/lhhcal17.htm].

12. "AARC Respiratory Therapist Human Resources Study—2000," *In the News,* Dec. 8, 2000. [http://www.aarc.org/headlines/resource_study/index.html].

13. U.S. Bureau of Labor Statistics, *Occupation Report: National Industry-Occupation Employment Matrix* (Washington, D.C.: U.S. Government Printing Office, Nov. 30, 1999). [ftp://ftp.bls.gov/pub/special.requests/ep/ind-occ.matrix//Occ0207_pdf/].

14. "Workplace Issues," *Profession @ a Glance,* Dec. 22, 2000. [http://www.asrt.org/profession_glance/workplace_issues.htm].

15. Christian Murray, "A Different Kind of Dental Loss: Shortage of New Dentists Is Starting to Worry Some Experts," *Morning Call* (Allentown, Pa.), Nov. 5, 2000. [http://www.mcall.com/html/health/front/dentistshortage.html].

16. "The Personnel File," *Modern HealthCare,* Apr. 2, 2001.

17. "Where Have All the Nurses Gone?" p. 5.

18. "Where Have All the Nurses Gone?" p. 3.

Chapter Nine

1. Barbara E. Tretheway and Jaye L. Martin, "Preventive Legislation, Gag Clauses Gasp Their Last Breath," *Minnesota Physicians* 10:12 (Mar. 1997): 28.

2. Tretheway and Martin, "Preventive Legislation," p. 28.

Chapter Ten

1. "Total Expenditure on Health—Per Capita, US$ PPP," in *OECD Health Data 2002,* 4th ed. (Paris: Organization for Economic Cooperation and Development, 2002). [http://www.oecd.org/xls/M00031000/M00031378.xls].

2. S. Heffler and others, "Health Spending Projections for 2001–2011: The Latest Outlook," *Health Affairs* (Mar.–Apr. 2002): 207–218.

3. U.S. Census Bureau, Table US-2001EST-01, "Time Series of National Population Estimates: April 1, 2000 to July 1, 2001" (Dec. 27, 2001). [http://eire.census.gov/popest/data/national/populartables/table01.php].

4. Centers for Medicare and Medicaid Services, Office of the Actuary, *The Nation's Health Dollar, CY 2000* (Baltimore, Md.: Centers for Medicare and Medicaid Services, June 2002). [http://cms.hhs.gov/charts/series].

5. "German Call for Radical Health Policy Change," *NewsEdge WorkGroups*, Apr. 20, 2001. [http://workgroups.newsedge.com/display_p.asp?doc_id=Nem0419600.5kl].

Chapter Twelve

1. Personal communication, Council of Accountable Physician Practices, Feb. 2003.

2. *Fast Facts on U.S. Hospitals from Hospital Statistics* (Chicago: American Hospital Association, Resource Center, Mar. 2001). [http://www.aha.org/esource/newpage.asp].

3. Institute for Clinical Systems Improvement, *2001 Annual Report,*p. 10.

4. HealthPartners, *HEDIS 2002 Report* (Minneapolis: HealthPartners, 2002). The report is based on dates of service for the year 2000.

5. Kaiser Permanente Performance Analysis Department, *HEDIS Performance Report* (Oakland, Calif.: Kaiser Permanente, 2002).

Chapter Fourteen

1. Gerard Anderson and James R. Knickman, "Changing the Chronic Care System to Meet People's Needs," *Health Affairs* 20 (Nov.–Dec. 2001): 146–160.

2. "Study Shows Weight Loss Can Cut Diabetes Risk," *Saint Paul Pioneer Press*, May 3, 2001, p. 5A.

3. HealthPartners Discover, *You Can Succeed at Weight Management* (Minneapolis, Minn.: HealthPartners Discover, Spring 2000).

4. Jill Burcum, "Your Health," *Star Tribune*, Oct. 10, 2000, P. E1.

5. David Chenoweth and Shellie Pfohl, "The High Cost of Couch Potatoes," *Business and Health* (Jan. 2000): 20–21.

6. Nico P. Pronk, *Economic Aspects of Obesity: A Managed Care Perspective* (Minneapolis, Minn.: HealthPartners Center for Health Promotion and HealthPartners Research Foundation, 2000).

7. Nico P. Pronk, *Population Health and Active Living: Economic Potential of Physical Activity Promotion* (Minneapolis, Minn.: HealthPartners Center for Health Promotion and HealthPartners Research Foundation, 2000).

8. "New NIH Minority Health Initiative." [http://www.raceandhealth. hhs.gov/sidebars/sbwhats17.htm].

9. Centers for Disease Control, National Center for Health Statistics, *Trends in Racial and Ethnic-Specific Rates for the Health Status Indicators: United States, 1990–98* (Washington, D.C.: U.S. Government Printing Office, Jan. 2002). Organization for Economic Cooperation and Development, *Health Data 2002* (Paris: Organization for Economic Cooperation and Development, 2002). [http://www.oecd.org/ EN/document/0,,EN-document-12-nodirectorate-no-1-29041– 12,00.html].

10. U.S. Department of Health and Human Services, "Goal 1— Eliminate Disparities in Infant Mortality Rates." [http://www. raceandhealth.hhs.gov/3rdpgBlue/Infant/3pgGoalsInfant.htm].

11. U.S. Department of Health and Human Services, "Goal 2— Eliminate Disparities in Cancer Screening and Management." [http://www.raceandhealth.hhs.gov/3rdpgBlue/Cancer/3pgGoals Cancer.htm].

12. Julie Bolen and others, "State-Specific Prevalence of Selected Health Behaviors, by Race and Ethnicity—Behavioral Risk Factor Surveillance System, 1997," *MMWR*, Mar. 24, 2000.

13. U.S. Department of Health and Human Services, "Goal 4— Eliminate Disparities in Diabetes." [http://www.raceandhealth.hhs. gov/3rdpgBlue/Diabetes/3pgGoalsDiabetes.htm].

14. U.S. Department of Health and Human Services, "Goal 5— Eliminate Disparities in HIV Infection/AIDS." [http://www. raceandhealth.hhs.gov/3rdpgBlue/HIV/3pgGoalsHIV.htm].

15. David Satcher, *Healthy People 2010* (Washington, D.C.: U.S. Department of Health and Human Services, 2000).

Chapter Fifteen

1. Jon B. Christianson, *Jockeying for Position: Specialist Strategies in Local Healthcare Markets* (Minneapolis: University of Minnesota, Feb. 2000).

Chapter Sixteen

1. Paul Frostin, *Sources of Health Insurance and Characteristics of the Uninsured: Analysis of the March 2002 Current Population Survey* (Washington, D.C.: Employee Benefit Research Institute, Dec. 2002).

2. Lisa Dubay, Ian Hill, and Genevieve Kenney, *Five Things Everyone Should Know About SCHIP* (Washington, D.C.: Urban Institute, Oct. 2002).

3. Emergency Medical Treatment and Active Labor Act, sec. 1867(a) of the Social Security Act, 42 USC 1395dd et seq.

4. Henry J. Kaiser Family Foundation, *Uninsured in America*, 2nd ed. (Menlo Park, Calif.: Kaiser Commission on Medicaid and the Uninsured, May 2000), p. 35.

5. Internal Revenue Service, Code of Federal Regulations (26), sec. 54.4980B-6, Question 1.

6. Sherry A. Glied, *Challenges and Options for Increasing the Number of Americans with Health Insurance* (New York: Commonwealth Fund, Jan. 2001), p. 5.

7. Conversation with Lynn Gruber, president, Minnesota Comprehensive Health Association.

8. Kaiser Family Foundation and Health Research and Educational Trust, "Employer Health Benefits: 2002 Annual Survey" (Menlo Park, Calif.: Kaiser Family Foundation, 2002).

Index